The Complete Guide to Becoming an Autism Friendly Professional

W0081224

Based on the award-winning *Autism Friendly Training Program*, created by the non-profit organization STARS for Autism, this book empowers the everyday professional to a better understanding and skill in working with, interacting with, serving, and teaching children and adults who have autism spectrum disorder (ASD).

After a thorough explanation of ASD and how it affects children, adults, families, and communities, this guide describes the *Autism Friendly Training Program* and gives the reader insight into what it means to become autism friendly and to be an autism friendly training presenter. This text will enable those who are neurotypical to gain insight into the person, the stories, and the lives of those with ASD. It is a guide to understand autism at a deeper level to enable relationship and support processes that define being autism friendly.

Providing the needed information, tools, and confidence to be autism friendly, this book will be beneficial to any and all businesses, organizations, groups, communities, families, and individuals who work with, serve, interact with, teach, parent, and experience life with an autistic person.

Robert Jason Grant, EdD, is a Licensed Professional Counselor, Advanced Certified Autism Specialist, and creator of AutPlay® Therapy. He serves on the Board of Directors for the Association for Play Therapy and is an accomplished autism author, advocate, and trainer.

Linda Barboa, PhD, has worked for several years as an educator in the United States and Europe. She has facilitated many autism trainings and is the author of several books about autism. She is currently the executive director of the nonprofit organization STARS for Autism.

Jan Luck holds a degree in Speech Pathology and Audiology. She is the board president for the nonprofit organization STARS for Autism. She is an author and advocate, and has trained hundreds of adults and children in the *Autism Friendly Training Program*.

Elizabeth Obrey is the vice president of STARS for Autism and currently works as a family advocate while pursuing a master's in Information Science and Learning Technologies. She is also a parent of children with multiple disabilities.

"The timely release of this book provides an accessible and informative appreciation of Autism Spectrum Disorder (ASD). With the rapid increase in recognition and diagnosis of children and adults with ASD, there has not been a better time to understand more about this condition and have tools to best support, encourage and welcome those who are neurodiverse among us, in all sectors of our community.

R. J. Grant, L. Barboa, J. Luck, and E. Obrey have written a sensitive account about autism that factors in the individual, family, groups, and organizations. It is a call to action, for not just mental health and education professionals that work with those with ASD, but also community leaders in all sectors, to build in systems to optimize function and contribution of those with ASD and to celebrate the strengths in our diverse communities that grow integrated, accepting, and flourishing societies."

Jacki Short, *counselling psychologist and Play Therapy supervisor, director of Sydney Centre for Creative Change in Sydney, Australia*

"As a practicing Speech-Language Pathologist, I highly recommend this book. It would be a great asset to parents, teachers, doctors, students, nurses, paraprofessionals, therapists, and family members. I wish I had this book as a guide 25 years ago, as I was entering the field of speech pathology. It really is that one book that has packed so many resources, stories, and easy to follow information into 10 chapters."

Marti Clark, *MS CCC-SLP*

"Parents of children with autism rally together to find professionals that will be an ally for them and a resource for their children's needs. When a professional is found that 'gets' our kiddos we share with other families who have children with autism. Being autism-friendly for a professional is a benefit and a gift for families who are already facing many obstacles for care. This book is a must-have for professionals who are willing to go that extra mile to meet the needs of those individuals and families impacted by autism."

Shelli Allen, *BS, "That Autism Mom", author, speaker, advocate*

"Written by knowledgeable and experienced professionals in the field of Autism Spectrum Disorder, this excellent and timely resource is an essential book that could impact how professionals relate to and interact with individuals on the spectrum, whether it be in the workplace or the social arena."

Renée Vajko Srch, *author of* Hope for Joshua *and* Miracle Moments

"Thank you for a thorough, accurate guide to understanding autism! I will be recommending this book to all my parents and to those who provide services to my students."

Brenda Bradshaw, *PhD, director of Infinity Academy*

"I recommend this book for all the teachers, parents, and all those who deal with people with autism day by day. And yes, for the people with autism as well. That way maybe the children and adults with autism will not feel they are 'weird' but just unique. It will help the teachers to understand the children, and the parents will see it is not their fault as many people say. It is a book that should be on the list of every teacher, school, and every house where someone with autism lives."

Els Speybrouck, *mum of Robin who has ASD, Harelbeke, Belgium*

"Kindness, compassion, understanding – these are all traits that make our world a better place. But humans are not cookie cutter and understanding individuals with autism can be tricky or confusing at times. Not anymore! After reading this guide, I feel prepared, informed, and *EXCITED* to advocate and implement strategies to make my profession, and myself, more Autism Friendly!"

Jen Hargove, *LPC, MAC, NBCC, owner, Hargrove Counseling LLC*

"From our first Autism Friendly Training to our proclamation signing, the Stars for Autism program has assisted our City, staff, and our citizens to become more aware of social engagement and environmental factors that affect those individuals on the autism spectrum. It is a fundamental training for our employees."

Renee Kingston, *Assistant City Administrator/City Clerk, City of Camdenton, Missouri*

"I have had the pleasure of reading the book *The Complete Guide to Becoming an Autism Friendly Professional*. This is a book that every business should have on hand for their employees to read to help them become an Autism Friendly Professional. It will help people to deal with an individual on the spectrum under different situations with appropriate responses."

Andrea Schultz, *owner/founder of Schultz's Tutoring and Playgroups*

"A refreshing book with wide and topical appeal, its in-depth understanding of autism will empower professionals and give them the confidence to engage positively with the autism community."

Stella Waterhouse, *author of* Autism Decoded

"As an attendee and guest speaker at an Autism Friendly Training, I highly recommend this book and program by the wonderful advocates of STARS for Autism."

Eli Winfrey, *autism advocate and president of Team Winfrey*

"Be aware; you have in your hands a powerful resource to make a difference and change lives. A necessary book for all of us who want to be fully equipped to educate, support, mentor, and include families on the autism spectrum. It's instructional, functional, and transformational. As you open this book, you get access to powerful resources that can make a difference and change lives."

Reverend Iromar Schreiber (aka Reverend Hugs), *LCMS pastor, Hope Lutheran Church*

"This is truly an amazing all-rounded book on autism! The book is full of tremendous information and insightful ideas that help the reader to get a better understanding and to see things from an autistic point of view. It also goes a step further to explain how you could be a responsible citizen to turn your community into an autism friendly place. The objective of the book is at an entirely different level and perspectives which is definitely a must-read for those who would like to know more about autism. I wholeheartedly believe that this book could help a lot of autistic children, adults, their parents and families, as well as professional practitioners in the field."

Canace Yee, *MA (Psych), RPT, APPTA, licensed trainer, Lego®-Based Therapy, founder and director, yNOTplay Play Therapy Hong Kong*

"This book is an invaluable tool for individuals working and interacting with people with autism. It is a professionally written and thorough resource guide for professionals and the general public, who want a better understanding of how autism affects the individual and how to help them in a manner that is useful and significant for them. From diagnosis to integration into the community, this book provides a step-by-step action plan on how communities and organizations can provide an autism friendly environment, allowing individuals with autism the opportunity to experience a positive interaction. This book provides professionals an insight into the world of autism and how every individual's experience is unique to them. The authors have provided a roadmap aimed at educating and bringing awareness to people who work and interact with individuals living with autism."

Linda Mastroianni, *Integration Aide/Special Care counselor*

"Yes! I'm so thrilled to see this book by this group of trusted professionals! Many professionals desire to be more Autism Friendly and this book can help you refine your strategies for success! Working alongside these authors for many years has taught me that their ideas come from a place of compassion and practicality. Now, they share their collective wisdom by offering tried and true strategies for your success! I highly recommend this read!"

Amy Stark Vaughan, *OTD, OTR/L, BCP, Doctor of Occupational Therapy, Board Certified in Pediatrics*

The Complete Guide to Becoming an Autism Friendly Professional

Working with Individuals, Groups, and Organizations

Robert Jason Grant, Linda Barboa, Jan Luck, and Elizabeth Obrey

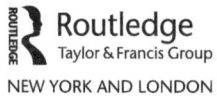

Routledge
Taylor & Francis Group

NEW YORK AND LONDON

First published 2022
by Routledge
605 Third Avenue, New York, NY 10158

and by Routledge
2 Park Square, Milton Park, Abingdon, Oxon OX14 4RN

Routledge is an imprint of the Taylor & Francis Group, an informa business

Library of Congress Cataloging-in-Publication Data
Names: Grant, Robert Jason, 1971- author. | Barboa, Linda, author. | Luck, Jan, author. | Obrey, Elizabeth, author.
Title: The complete guide to becoming an autism friendly professional : working with individuals, groups, and organizations / Robert Jason Grant, Linda Barboa, Jan Luck, Elizabeth Obrey.
Description: New York, NY : Routledge, 2021. | Includes bibliographical references and index. | Summary: "Based on the award-winning Autism Friendly Training
Identifiers: LCCN 2020055471 (print) | LCCN 2020055472 (ebook) | ISBN 9780367615895 (hardback) | ISBN 9780367615888 (paperback) | ISBN 9781003105633 (ebook)
Subjects: LCSH: Autism spectrum disorders--Patients--Care. | Employees--Training of.
Classification: LCC RC553.A88 G745 2021 (print) | LCC RC553.A88 (ebook) | DDC 616.85/8820023--dc23
LC record available at https://lccn.loc.gov/2020055471
LC ebook record available at https://lccn.loc.gov/2020055472

ISBN: 978-0-367-61589-5 (hbk)
ISBN: 978-0-367-61588-8 (pbk)
ISBN: 978-1-003-10563-3 (ebk)

DOI: 10.4324/9781003105633

Typeset in Times New Roman
by Taylor & Francis Books

Contents

Illustrations

Acknowledgments

Thank you to STARS for Autism and all the work they have done through the years to create and promote the *Autism Friendly Training Program.* Thank you to my coauthors – Linda, Jan, and Elizabeth – you all inspire me with your passion for serving the autism community and we make a great team! I also want to thank all the individuals who have completed an *Autism Friendly Training* throughout the years – thank you for your dedication to improving experiences for those with autism.

Dr. Robert Jason Grant

I would like to acknowledge the City of Battlefield, Missouri for their forward-thinking acceptance of the Autism Friendly Program. The excellence they displayed in becoming the first Officially Autism Friendly City in Missouri served as a model for other communities. Through the implementation of this project, the City of Battlefield was honored with the "Most Innovative Project" by the State of Missouri, bringing recognition to the program. I extend our thanks to the Mayor, the Police Department, the Advisory Park Board, the Board of Aldermen, and the citizens for their support of the Autism Friendly Program.

Dr. Linda Barboa

I would like to thank the STARS for Autism volunteers for their many hours of dedicated service. They have attended presentations, manned information booths, set up venues, chaired meetings, helped other volunteers, presented information to others, and given of themselves in so many ways. None of this would be possible without their heartfelt dedication to increasing awareness and acceptance of those on the autism spectrum.

Jan Luck

I would like to honor all of the first responders who participate in the STARS for Autism trainings as I cherish the stories of success and challenges they share year after year. Accepting that knowledge is power, they have gone above and beyond to serve those diagnosed with autism and their families while keeping our communities safe and friendly.

Elizabeth Obrey

All the authors wish to acknowledge Mr. Landon Kemp for his contribution of engaging illustrations which serve to bring the book concepts to life. His drawings promote understanding and retention of the material presented, and for that we are thankful for his talents and generosity. The authors also wish to thank all those who reviewed our book and provided endorsements – we are incredibly grateful for the time you took to share your thoughts. And finally, we would like to thank Dr. Stephen Shore for providing a wonderful foreword for our book!

Foreword

Autism Friendly is a relatively new term in the autism community. At the forefront of the *Autism Friendly* movement, the Complete *Guide to Becoming an Autism Friendly Professional* reframes how professionals and others can support autistic individuals in leading fulfilling and productive lives. Rather than working against the characteristics of autism and making the person "less autistic," focus turns towards understanding and working *with* the characteristics and implementing environmental modifications as needed to empower all parties towards greater mutual understanding and promoting success in education, employment, and in the community at large.

A vital part of the *Autism Friendly* movement requires authentic and meaningful involvement and participation of autistic individuals on all aspects of life pertaining to autism; be it education, employment, modification of the environment, and research. Through this book, Grant, Barboa, Luck, and Obrey (the authors) expertly model meaningful and authentic involvement by including numerous voices of autistic individuals to validate the points made in the book. The common thread presented by the autistic voices employed in this book of being misunderstood in a confusing world is combined with impactful insights from these same individuals and the authors on how things could have, and can be made better for everyone.

Relatedly, in my international travels educating teachers, places of employment, first responders, police departments, and others, I find increasing numbers of people report that their work done in preparing their part of the world to be autistic friendly makes them better overall at what they do. For example, educators commonly tell me that once they understand and integrate their mindset for meaningful involvement of their autistic students, they become better overall teachers for all of their students. Similarly, increasing numbers of supervisors indicate that they become better communicators and managers as they engage in the process of successfully including their autistic employees as equals.

While the concept of *autism friendly* did not exist during my time as a student from pre-school through my doctoral studies, nor in the workplace, I feel we are in a very exciting time where autistics and others in the neurodiverse community are being welcomed and valued for who we are and what we *can* do rather being thought of as a poor imitation of a person not on the autism spectrum. *The Complete Guide to Becoming an Autism Friendly Professional* is another step in moving neurodiverse values forward and a welcome addition to the family of autism related literature.

Stephen Mark Shore, EdD, internationally known educator, writer, consultant, and presenter on issues related to autism

Introduction

What is autism? It is easy to find many definitions of the term, descriptions of the disorder, and diagnostic procedures. Symptomology, presentation, and manifestations are clearly outlined in many resources (many will be covered in this book). But our technical knowledge of autism spectrum disorder (ASD) is only the beginning of what is autism. It tells us something but arguably not the most important parts to what is autism. A more holistic view suggests that autism not be viewed as simply a definition, but instead as a person. At least, it is a person who receives the diagnosis, who lives with the manifestations, who experiences the symptomology, and who navigates autism in the various domains that make up their life. Selfe (2013) explained that autism is a complex condition. The variation between individuals along the spectrum and co-occurrence of other issues adds to this complexity. Those with ASD are complex and although we require definitions for common understanding, it is important to begin any journey of understanding autism by acknowledging there are many people, navigating life in many ways, who are connected to this term.

Among the many considerations about autism is that it can create needs in the ability to relate to other human beings, inability to make friendships, difficulty understanding others, and challenges participating in society meaningfully and independently. Communication and sensory challenges amplify the difficulties and can created social isolation leaving an autistic individual to retreat into their own world (Selfe, 2013). As if this were not enough, autistic individuals must survive in communities where the term "special needs" is playground slang for "retarded," where dysregulated meltdowns and panic attacks are viewed as tantrums, where disability benefits and insurance are assumed by many to be associated with welfare moochers, where celebrities, politicians, and political pundits use the term autistic as a derogatory and biting insult to those they do not like, and where parents are judged, accused, and insulted on a regular basis because of opinions about their child's behavior in public.

A mother recalled a story of being in a restaurant with her autistic son and neurotypical daughter. They were thrilled as this was the first time they had been able to successfully get him to participate in going to a

DOI: 10.4324/9781003105633-1

restaurant. As they were sitting at their table, he was being noticeably loud and due to his anxieties was being obsessive about several details with the table, the menu, and the waitress. The mother was doing her best to guide him through, and the waitress was kind and patient. Considering his history and the struggles that he historically demonstrated, this restaurant outing was a nice improvement and showed good progress. Toward the end of their dining experience, a man who had been sitting nearby was done with his meal and, as he was leaving, stopped at the family's table. He proceeded to tell the mother that she "Needed to get control of that damn brat and teach him some manners." He further directed to the mother "Maybe you are the problem and need your damn face slapped." He then angrily left the restaurant. The joys of their first fairly successful restaurant experience were crushed, the child's anxiety, which had progressively diminishing during the dining experience had now rocketed up, and the family had to quickly leave the restaurant. If there were an example of how to NOT be autism friendly, this man would certainly be our guide. Unfortunately, this man is a man, woman, child, business, policy, etc. in every community and in so many experiences for autistic individuals.

In 2013, a group of individuals passionate about autism came together with a goal to be part of the solution to provide education and awareness to others about autism. They desired to be a part of ending the stigma and struggles that those with ASD encounter on a daily basis. They created a book titled *Stars in Her Eyes: Navigating the Maze of Childhood Autism.* Dr. Linda Barboa and Elizabeth Obrey, with contributions from Shelli Allen, Sandy Nicholson and Jan Luck, collaborated to create a resource that would help families navigate the complex world of autism. Prior to the creation of this book, Dr. Barboa was the director of a school for children with autism spectrum disorder. She spent much of her time sharing information with parents of newly diagnosed ASD children. Parents were overwhelmed with information and were looking for simple, understandable, and relatable information to help their child.

Dr. Barboa decided the best way to present the much-needed information was to gather a group of individuals with different backgrounds and knowledge of autism to each give their unique perspective on different aspects of autism and compile that information into a positive reader-friendly book. She asked two well-respected parents of autistic children, a public-school speech therapist and a classroom teacher, to help present the information in book form. After the book was published, the group began to receive requests to speak to organizations about increasing acceptance and awareness of autism. This was the beginning of STARS (Service, Training, Awareness, Respect, Support) for Autism, a 501c3 organization (a particular nonprofit organization that has been approved by the Internal Revenue Service as a tax-exempt, charitable organization) based in Southwest Missouri.

STARS for Autism was established to provide autism education and training to individuals, groups, organizations, and communities. Among the group's endeavors was included the organization of the "Autism Information Blast," a large yearly event that showcases autism resources, business, and products to the general public. They also worked with several cities to help them become an *Autism Friendly City*, which followed their Missouri Municipal League Innovation Award winning program. They also partnered with local businesses and schools in Pekin, Illinois to present information and distribute *Albert is My Friend: Helping Children Understand Autism* to grade school children. The nonprofit organization regularly strategized how to best meet the training needs of individuals and groups and as a result, the *Autism Friendly Training* was created and has become a highly valued and sought-after resource.

This award-winning training is typically promoted as a full-day training which allows attendees to understand what autism is and how to interact with those on the autism spectrum. This training promotes awareness of the social, sensory, and environmental barriers which affect individuals who have autism. It is designed for educators, therapists, government employees, and professionals across a variety of settings, to gain valuable information for working with, serving, and interacting with autistic individuals. This training provides a valuable resource for anyone in any setting to better understand and interact with those with autism spectrum disorder. The *Autism Friendly Training* has been adapted to different lengths and modified to focus on specific groups such as first responders and educators. In 2019, STARS partnered with AutPlay® Therapy to offer the *Autism Friendly Training* in an online/home study format and to develop other derivatives (described later in this book) of the basic *Autism Friendly Training*.

To date, thousands of individuals, including law enforcement personnel, fire fighters, EMTs, teachers, volunteers, business owners, mental health therapists, families, and others wanting to know more about autism and becoming autism friendly have been trained through this program. The program continues to grow and reach new audiences around the world. The latest achievement is the construction of this book, which highlights the *Autism Friendly Training* and all its derivatives. This book provides easy access for individuals around the globe to learn about and understand what it means to be autism friendly.

This book begins by presenting information about autism and how it affects children, adults, families, and communities. It further describes the *Autism Friendly Training Program* and gives the reader insight into what it means to become autism friendly, complete an *Autism Friendly Training*, and to become an autism friendly training presenter. This book is also a journey for those who are neurotypical to gain insight into the person, the stories, and the lives of autistic individuals. It is a guide to understanding autism at a deeper level to enable relationship and support processes that define being autism friendly. Businesses, organizations, groups, communities, families, and individuals who work with, serve, interact with, teach, parent, and experience life with someone with ASD will find the material in this book targets you – giving you the needed information, tools, and confidence to make a positive impact in the life of an autistic person by your commitment to becoming autism friendly. The authors would like to note that language has been varied throughout the book to respect different views in the autism community. Terms such as autistic person (identity first language), person with autism (person first language), disability, and differently abled have been interchanged throughout the book. The authors fully support neurodiversity affirming and informed processes when interacting with autistic individuals. Neurodiversity affirming is defined as recognizing neural and biological differences and understanding that not every brain works the same. Each individual may experience the world very differently and differences are not wrong or bad but valued.

1 About Autism

Research, writings, and trainings abound about autism spectrum disorder (ASD), yet many individuals are vastly unaware of what ASD is and how it affects children, adults, families, and communities. Having information easily accessible about ASD provides the opportunity for the lay person to advance their knowledge of autism and be more effective in parenting, working with, and serving those with ASD, and ultimately becoming autism friendly.

The Autism Society of America (2020) described ASD as a complex developmental disability with signs typically appearing during early childhood. ASD affects a person's ability to communicate and interact with others. ASD is defined by a certain set of behaviors and is a "spectrum condition" that affects individuals differently and to varying degrees. There is no known single cause of autism, but increased awareness and early diagnosis with intervention and access to appropriate services lead to significantly improved outcomes. Some of the behaviors associated with autism include delayed learning of language; difficulty engaging or holding a conversation; difficulty with executive functioning, which relates to reasoning and planning; narrow, intense interests; poor motor skills and sensory sensitivities.

The Centers for Disease Control and Prevention (CDC) (2020) proposed that ASD is a developmental disability that can cause significant social, communication, and behavioral challenges. There is often nothing about how autistic people look that sets them apart from other people, but autistic individuals may communicate, interact, behave, and learn in ways that are different from most other people. The learning, thinking, and problem-solving abilities of people with ASD can range from severely challenged to gifted. Some people with autism require a great deal of help in their daily lives; others need far less. A diagnosis of ASD now includes several conditions that used to be diagnosed separately: autistic disorder, pervasive developmental disorder not otherwise specified (PDD-NOS), and Asperger's syndrome. These conditions are now all called autism spectrum disorder.

Monteiro (2016) proposed that autistic individuals display a pattern of differences in their development, or style, that affects the way they use language and communicate with others; how they understand and participate in

DOI: 10.4324/9781003105633-2

social relationships; the way in which they understand, manage, and regulate emotions; and how they respond to and manage sensory input and preferred areas of interest. Autism can affect an individual in a myriad of ways with social, emotional, motor, developmental, and learning deficits all being present. For those interacting with autistic individuals, it is essential to possess accurate information in order to understand the level of impairment and equally understand the existing skill strengths of the individual.

Autism ranges from mild to severe in terms of impairment on an individual. An individual on the mild end of the spectrum may be able to function without regard in a school, work, or independent living setting and eventually reach a point where they no longer meet the criteria for ASD. An individual on the severe end of the spectrum may be unable to speak and have more serious developmental delays. Even if two individuals have the same diagnosis, no two individuals with autism are alike. One person with ASD may be nonverbal and have a low IQ, while another person with the same diagnosis may have an above average IQ, and yet a third person may be verbally and intellectually precocious. Moreover, often labeling terms "low functioning" and "high functioning" were historically used to describe the person's placement on the autism spectrum (Exkorn, 2005) and not a reflection that there are only two categories of autism presentation.

A more accurate way to view the spectrum of autism would be to view each person individually and assess each person, plotting them where they currently place in each developmental area. Because, in fact, autistic individuals do not fall into one of two categories – low or high functioning; each person has their own place on the spectrum according to their individual presentation and skill level (Grant 2017a). Because of the range of manifestation and the myriad of issues that can accompany autism, it is essential that those involved take into account the individual and align their views to address the individual's particular skill needs, strengths, and issues. Do not make assumptions about a person because they have autism. The diagnosis alone does not tell you about them or how the autism affects their life.

Common Presentations in ASD

Several terms exist that are common language related to autism and help define some of the more present features of those with autism. The following terms and definitions are adapted from the National Institute of Mental Health (2020) and Autism Speaks (2020). A complete list of terms related to ASD can be found in Appendix 1.

Ableism – Discrimination in favor of able-bodied people. The belief that those without a disability or disorder are superior and there is something flawed and wrong with those who do, and they do not deserve equal thought or treatment.

Atypical – A term that means not typical, or not conforming to the common type: irregular or abnormal.

Neurotypical – A label for people who are not on the autism spectrum; specifically, neurotypical people have neurological development and states that are consistent with what most people would perceive as typical development.

Compulsions – The deliberate repetitive behaviors that follow specific rules, such as pertaining to cleaning, checking, or counting. In young children, restricted patterns of interest may be an early sign of compulsions.

Developmental delay – When a child does not reach his or her developmental milestones at the expected times. It is an ongoing major or minor delay in the process of development.

Dysregulation struggles – Dysregulation is a term used in the mental health community to refer to an emotional response that is poorly modulated and does not fall within the conventionally accepted range of emotive response. It can be looked at as a person's inability to manage or regulate their emotions which typically results in various negative behaviors.

Echolalia – An individual's automatic repetition of vocalizations made by another person. It is closely related to echopraxia, the automatic repetition of movements made by another person. Echolalia can be present with autism and other developmental disabilities. A typical presentation of echolalia might be as follows: A person is asked "Do you want dinner?"; the person echoes back "Do you want dinner?" followed by a pause, and possibly then a response, "Yes. What's for dinner?" In delayed echolalia, a phrase is repeated after a delay, such as a person with autism who repeats TV commercials, favorite movie scripts, or parental reprimands.

Emotional regulation struggles – Emotional regulation is an individual's ability to notice and respond to internal and external input that elicits an emotion, and then adjust their emotions and behavior to the demands of their surroundings. Emotional regulation is the ability to recognize feelings, understand what is creating the feeling, and understand how to appropriately express or manage the feeling. This can often be a struggle area for those with ASD.

Eye gaze – Looking at the face of others to check and see what they are looking at and to signal interest in interacting. It is a nonverbal behavior used to convey or exchange information or express emotions without the use of words, which is often a struggle area for autistic individuals.

Hyperarousal – A state of increased psychological and physiological tension marked by such effects as reduced pain tolerance, anxiety, exaggerated startle responses, insomnia, and fatigue.

Hyperlexia – Characterized by having an average or above average IQ and word-reading ability well above what would be expected at a given age. It can be viewed as a super ability in which word recognition ability goes far above expected levels of skill.

Hypoarousal – A physiological state where your body slows down. It may include feelings of sadness, irritability, and nervousness.

Individualized Education Program (IEP) – An educational plan designed to meet the unique education needs of one child, who may have a disability, as defined by federal regulations. An IEP is intended to help children reach targeted educational goals. IEPs are mandated by the Individuals with Disabilities Education Act (IDEA).

Joint attention – The shared focus of two individuals on an object. It is achieved when one individual alerts another to an object by means of eye-gazing, pointing, or other verbal or nonverbal indication. An individual gazes at another individual, points to an object and then returns their gaze to the individual.

Obsessions – The domination of one's thoughts or feelings by a persistent idea, image, desire, etc. Obsessions are thoughts that reoccur and persist despite efforts to ignore or confront them.

Perseverating behaviors – Refers to repeating or "getting stuck" carrying out a behavior, a thought, verbalization, etc. (e.g., putting in and taking out a puzzle piece) when it is no longer appropriate.

Pragmatic speech issues – Refers to language used to communicate and socialize. It is social language skills that we use in our daily interactions with others. This includes what we say, how we say it, our nonverbal communication (eye contact, facial expressions, body language etc.) and how appropriate our interactions are in a given situation.

Receptive language issues – The comprehension of language; listening and understanding what is communicated. It is the receiving aspect of language. Sometimes, reading is included when referring to receptive language, but some use the term for spoken communication only. It involves being attentive to what is said, the ability to comprehend the message, the speed of processing the message, and concentrating on the message. Receptive language also includes understanding figurative language, as well as literal language. Receptive language includes being able to follow a series of commands.

Sensory processing struggles – Sensory processing is the way the nervous system receives messages from the senses and turns them into appropriate motor and behavioral responses. Processing issues exist when sensory signals do not get organized into appropriate responses which create challenges in performing everyday tasks and may manifest in motor clumsiness, behavioral problems, anxiety, depression, and school failure. The eight sensory areas are sight, smell, taste, hearing, touch, vestibular, proprioception, and interoception.

Social reciprocity struggles – Challenges in the back-and-forth flow of social interaction. The term reciprocity refers to how the behavior of one person influences and is influenced by the behavior of another person and vice versa.

Spectrum disorder – A term that refers to three disorders that previously existed using the Diagnostic and Statistical Manual (DSM-IV) which included autistic disorder, Asperger's syndrome, and pervasive developmental disorder NOS.

Stimming behavior – A repetitive body movement, such as hand flapping, that is hypothesized to stimulate one or more senses. The term is shorthand for self-stimulation. It is repetitive movement, or stereotypy, is often referred to as stimming under the hypothesis that it has a function related to sensory input. Stimming only creates an issue as it could bother those observing the stimming. For those with ASD, stimming can be a self-soothing experience.

Theory of mind – The ability to attribute mental states (beliefs, intents, desires, pretending, knowledge) to oneself and others and to understand that others have beliefs, desires, and intentions that are different from one's own.

ASD Strengths and Abilities

Autistic Individuals can possess the same strengths and talents found in any neurotypical person and often possess unique strengths and abilities due to being autistic. ASD individuals often have challenges to overcome in building routines and relationships that are functional and fulfilling and while much of current research and therapeutic intervention focuses on addressing those challenges, a growing amount of research is showing that people living with ASD may also benefit from unique strengths previously unnoticed by the general population. Those involved and working with individuals with autism should focus on each person and their individual areas of strength and growth, as well as the personality qualities that set them apart and make them unique. The more that is understood about how a person with ASD's brain is organized differently from a neurotypical brain, the more awareness is gained that a different way of organizing can be valued (Panzano, 2018).

The variety and type of skills and abilities that seem to coincide with ASD are many. Certainly, each autistic person will possess their own set of skills and strengths that can be highlighted and used successfully in a variety of setting and interactions. Table 1.1 illustrates some of the more commons strengths and abilities found in those with ASD.

Statistical Awareness of ASD in the United States

Statistical information about autism spectrum disorder from the Centers for Disease Control and Prevention (2020).

- It is estimated that an average of 1 in 54 children in the United States have ASD.
- Autism is reported to occur in all racial, ethnic, and socioeconomic groups.
- Autism is almost four times more common among boys.

Table 1.1 Common Strengths and Abilities Found in ASD

Learning to read at an early age (hyperlexia)
Advanced expressive language skills
String visual learners (visual memory recall)
Concrete and logical thinking
Good with schedules, routines, and consistency
Precise and detail orientated
Exceptional honesty and reliability
Follow rules and policies with efficiency
Have an excellent sense of direction
Very punctual
Able to concentrate (single-minded focus)

- About 1 in 6 (17%) children aged 3–17 years were diagnosed with a developmental disability, as reported by parents, during a study period of 2009–2017. These included autism, attention-deficit/hyperactivity disorder, blindness, and cerebral palsy, among others.
- Autism tends to occur more often in people who have certain genetic or chromosomal conditions. About 10% of children with autism are also identified as having Down Syndrome, Fragile X Syndrome, Tuberous Sclerosis, and other genetic and chromosomal disorders.
- ASD commonly co-occurs with other developmental, psychiatric, neurologic, chromosomal, and genetic diagnoses. The co-occurrence of one or more non-ASD developmental diagnoses is 83%. The co-occurrence of one or more psychiatric diagnoses is 10%.
- About 40% of children with ASD do not speak at all. Another 25%–30% of children with autism have some words at 12 to 18 months of age and then lose them. Other children with ASD may speak but not until later in childhood.
- Almost half (46%) of those identified with autism have average to above average intellectual ability.
- The median age of earliest ASD diagnosis is between 4.5 and 5.5 years, but for 51–91 percent of children with an ASD, developmental concerns had been recorded before three years of age.
- Research has shown that a diagnosis of autism at 18 months can be reliable, valid, and stable. Despite evidence that ASD can often be identified at around 18 months, many children do not receive final diagnoses until they are much older.
- Studies have shown that many parents of children with ASD notice a developmental problem before their child's first birthday. Concerns about vision and hearing were more often reported in the first year, and differences in social, communication, and fine motor skills were evident from six months of age.

- It is estimated to cost at least $17,000 more per year to care for a child with autism compared to a child without ASD. Costs include health care, education, ASD-related therapy, family-coordinated services, and caregiver time. For a child with more severe ASD, costs per year increase to over $21,000. Taken together, it is estimated that total societal costs of caring for children with autism were over $9 billion in 2011.

Diagnosis of ASD

Autism spectrum disorder is an American Psychiatric Association Diagnostic and Statistical Manual 5th Edition (American Psychiatric Association, 2014) diagnosis that is usually given after a thorough psychological evaluation; wherein, the evaluator measures the child or adolescent's behavior across a myriad of tests, assessments, and observations. The disorder is a spectrum disorder meaning the symptoms vary in intensity from severe to very mild. Common terms used to describe the variance include low and high functioning, or severe to mild impairment.

A synopsis of the Diagnostic and Statistical Manual 5th Edition (2014) criteria for receiving an ASD diagnosis is presented below:

A. Persistent deficits in social communication and social interaction across multiple contexts, as manifested by the following, currently or by history:

   1. Deficits in social-emotional reciprocity, ranging, for example, from abnormal social approach and failure of normal back-and-forth conversation; to reduced sharing of interests, emotions, or affect; to failure to initiate or respond to social interactions.
   2. Deficits in nonverbal communicative behaviors used for social interaction, ranging, for example, from poorly integrated verbal and nonverbal communication; to abnormalities in eye contact and body language or deficits in understanding and use of gestures; to a total lack of facial expressions and nonverbal communication.
   3. Deficits in developing, maintaining, and understanding relationships, ranging, for example, from difficulties adjusting behavior to suit various social contexts; to difficulties in sharing imaginative play or in making friends; to absence of interest in peers.

B. Restricted, repetitive patterns of behavior, interests, or activities, as manifested by at least two of the following, currently or by history:

   1. Stereotyped or repetitive motor movements, use of objects, or speech (e.g., simple motor stereotypies, lining up toys or flipping objects, echolalia, idiosyncratic phrases).

2. Insistence on sameness, inflexible adherence to routines, or ritualized patterns of verbal or nonverbal behavior (e.g., extreme distress at small changes, difficulties with transitions, rigid thinking patterns, greeting rituals, need to take same route or eat same food every day).
3. Highly restricted, fixated interests that are abnormal in intensity or focus (e.g., strong attachment to or preoccupation with unusual objects, excessively circumscribed or perseverative interest).
4. Hyper- or hyporeactivity to sensory input or unusual interests in sensory aspects of the environment (e.g., apparent indifference to pain/temperature, adverse response to specific sounds or textures, excessive smelling or touching of objects, visual fascination with lights or movement).

C. Symptoms must be present in the early developmental period (but may not become fully manifest until social demands exceed limited capacities or may be masked by learned strategies in later life).
D. Symptoms cause clinically significant impairment in social, occupational, or other important areas of current functioning.
E. These disturbances are not better explained by intellectual disability (intellectual developmental disorder) or global developmental delay. Intellectual disability and autism spectrum disorder frequently co-occur; to make comorbid diagnoses of autism spectrum disorder and intellectual disability, social communication should be below that expected for general developmental level.

The DSM 5 Levels of Support for ASD Diagnosis

Level 3: Requiring Very Substantial Support – Severe deficits in verbal and nonverbal social communication skills cause severe impairments in functioning, very limited initiation of social interactions, and minimal response to social overtures from others. For example, a person with few words of intelligible speech who rarely initiates interaction and, when they do, makes unusual approaches to meet needs only and responds to only very direct social approaches. Inflexibility of behavior, extreme difficulty coping with change, or other restricted/repetitive behaviors markedly interfere with functioning in all spheres. Great distress/difficulty changing focus or action.

Level 2: Requiring Substantial Support – Marked deficits in verbal and nonverbal social communication skills; social impairments apparent even with supports in place; limited initiation of social interactions; and reduced or abnormal responses to social overtures from others. For example, a person who speaks in simple sentences, whose interaction is limited to narrow special interests, and who has markedly odd nonverbal communication. Inflexibility of behavior, difficulty coping with change, or other restricted/repetitive behaviors appear frequently enough to be obvious to the casual observer and interfere with functioning in a variety of contexts. Distress and/or difficulty changing focus or action.

Level 1: Requiring Support – Without supports in place, deficits in social communication cause noticeable impairments. Difficulty initiating social interactions and clear examples of atypical or unsuccessful responses to social overtures of others. May appear to have decreased interest in social interactions. For example, a person who can speak in full sentences and engages in communication but whose to-and-fro conversation with others fails, and whose attempts to make friends are odd and typically unsuccessful. Inflexibility of behavior causes significant interference with functioning in one or more contexts. Difficulty switching between activities. Problems of organization and planning hamper independence.

Diagnosis of autism is typically done through a thorough psychological evaluation conducted by a trained psychologist which would be a medical diagnosis. Schools may also implement testing to diagnose for ASD which would be an educational diagnosis. Psychiatrists, neurologists, and medical doctors are also capable of providing a medical autism diagnosis. The most thorough, unbiased, and quantitative process for diagnosing ASD is having the child participate in a psychological evaluation. This process typically includes several assessment/evaluation inventories and the process can take anywhere from three hours to two days to complete.

There are two inventories used to diagnose ASD that are considered gold standard inventories. Gold standard meaning these inventories have validity and reliability measures to produce the best most accurate assessment for diagnosis. The two inventories for autism that are considered gold standard are the Autism Diagnostic Observation Schedule (ADOS) and the Autism Diagnostic Interview – Revised (ADI-R). Other popular inventories may be used as well such as the Childhood Autism Rating Scale (CARS). It is considered that a reliable and accurate diagnosis of ASD can be acquired as early as 18 months of age. Many individuals with ASD do not receive a diagnosis at 18 months of age; most diagnosis of ASD occurs between the ages of 4.5 and 5.5. The earlier the diagnosis, the earlier treatment can begin, and early intervention with ASD has produced the best research outcomes for gains in skill and functioning ability (Grant, 2018a).

Grant (2020) stated that beyond the criteria outlined to receive an ASD diagnosis, children and adolescents with autism typically have additional skill needs and developmental issues. Splintered skill development is one manifestation that is common in children with developmental disorders. Splinter skills are abilities that are disconnected from their usual context or are very specific abilities that do not generalize to other capabilities. Because they are just a "splinter," or fraction, of a meaningful set of skills, splinter skills may not be particularly useful in real-world situations.

Examples include the ability to memorize a bus schedule without understanding how to get to a bus station or buy a ticket. Another example is being able to memorize a multiplication table but not being able to complete a multiplication question on a math test.

Autistic children may display uneven development. A child with ASD may be at a developmental level far beyond their chronological age in one area of development and at the same time, far below their chronological age in another area of development. For example, a nine-year old child with autism may have expressive language ability at an adult level (well beyond their chronological age) but have emotional regulation ability at a preschool aged level (well below their chronological age).

Causes of Autism

Chasen (2014) stated that professionals in the field of autism continue to explore and debate possible causes of autism. Even though there is no scientifically validated cause, there are multiple theories. With no one theory being clearly conclusive, it seems reasonable to assume that some of the causes of autism, and increasing rates of diagnoses, are a result of multiple or a combination of factors. These factors may include abnormalities in brain structure or function; genetic influences; problems during pregnancy or delivery; and environmental factors such as viral infections, metabolic imbalances, and exposure to chemicals.

Autism is considered a lifelong condition. Many individuals with significant impairment as a child gained skills and have presented as adults with little to no impairment. This type of process is not unusual and is desired and the focal point of many ASD treatments or therapies. Although this does happen, it does not mean the individual has been cured of their autism or that they are no longer autistic. The impact the ASD has on an individual can certainly change (even dramatically) throughout their lifetime but change does not negate the predominant view that autism is a lifelong condition.

When discussing the cause of ASD and viewing autism as a lifelong condition, it is important to discuss the construct of neurodiversity. The term neurodiversity was first used by Judy Singer, an Australian social scientist, herself autistic, and first appeared in print in the *Atlantic* in 1998. Neurodiversity is the concept that humans do not come in a one-size-fits-all neurologically "normal" package. Instead, it recognizes that all variations of human neurological function need to be respected as just another way of being, and that neurological differences like autism are the result of normal/natural variations in the human genome. Neurodiversity is seen as a movement by many towards more equal treatment and more widespread acceptance for those on the spectrum, and with disabilities in general. The idea is that if autism is seen as a normal variation of the human experience, then autistic people will be treated more humanely and with more understanding. It encourages others to appreciate that those with ASD might have different needs or different ways of coping and this is acceptable. Rather than trying to bend someone with autism into a definition of "normal" behaviors, society might bend to allow for differences in behavior and needs, and create more opportunities for inclusion in schools, workplaces, etc. (Bennie, 2016).

The concept of neurodiversity is most especially important to those with ASD who have intact language and no learning difficulties such that they can self-advocate. Indeed, these individuals with autism can function independently and may even "pass" as neurotypical. They advocate for their way of processing, discerning, socializing, and viewing the world as a diverse strength that should be valued not pathologized and looked at as needing to change. There are also those who, while embracing some aspects of the concept of neurodiversity as applied to autism, argue that the severe challenges faced by many autistic people fit better within a more classical medical model. Many of these are parents of autistic children or autistic individuals who struggle substantially in any environment, who may have almost no language, exhibit severe learning difficulties, suffer gastrointestinal pain or epilepsy, appear to be in anguish for no apparent reason or lash out against themselves or others. Many of those who adopt the medical model of autism call for prevention and cure of the serious impairments that can be associated with ASD. In contrast, those who support neurodiversity see such language as a threat to autistic people's existence, no different than eugenics (Baron-Cohen, 2019).

There is a valid argument for all of the terms "disorder," "disability," "difference" and "disease" being applicable to different forms of autism or to the co-occurring conditions that can often exist with ASD. Neurodiversity is a valid cause for the autism community; our brains are all different and this should be valued and appreciated. Neurodiversity as a movement of diversity acceptance can be supported while still supporting that some with autism fall under a more medical model of treatment. It is likely that those who work with, serve, and interact with autistic individuals will encounter different opinions regarding terminology they prefer. Some may advocate for person first language (person with autism), while others may want to be called an autistic person. Some may prefer the term disability while others prefer differently abled. The autism friendly professional will take care to ask the person what they prefer and honor their preference.

Therapy and ASD

There exists a significant number of purported autism focused treatments/ therapies. Many of the most recognized and evidence-based treatments consist of behavioral methods, social skills training, and developmental approaches. There also exist bio-medical and existential approaches. Siri and Lyons (2010) suggested that since the etiology as well as the manifestations of ASD are influenced by a variety of multiple factors, a one-size-fits all approach to therapy and intervention is not the most beneficial approach. No two individuals will respond to the same combination of therapies. Each person's therapy plan needs to be unique, taking into consideration the specific symptoms the individual exhibits, the results of tests administered, and observations of the person. Many individuals with autism participate in some type of skill development intervention. The variety and depth of the skill intervention can look different for each person, but most current evidence-based treatment approaches for ASD involve some type of skill development component.

It would be easy to produce a list of over 100 promoted and advertised therapies for ASD. Promoted treatments include biomedical, behavioral, developmental, alternative, and difficult to categorize interventions. With the variety of options regarding autism therapies, and considering the vulnerability issues many individuals struggle with in searching for a therapy that will help improve their needs, it becomes important to critically evaluate promoted ASD therapy. Grant (2018a) proposed the following guide to serve as a protocol for evaluating an autism treatment/therapy.

1. What does the research say about the promoted ASD focused therapy? Is there any research support? Is the therapy an evidence-based or promising therapy for ASD needs? Does the treatment incorporate any evidence-based practices? A therapy approach may be helpful even if it is not evidence-based, but it is important to know what research has been presented on the treatment approach.
2. What are the potential risks of participating in the therapy? Are there any potentially dangerous side effects? Can any harm be done to the individual? Is the therapy affirming of the person and not devaluing of them or their autism? If a treatment approach contains possible harm or risk to the individual, it should be highly scrutinized before beginning.
3. What is the cost of the therapy? How much money will the person have to pay out of pocket to receive the treatment? It is important to be aware that some treatments may exist to take advantage of those with ASD. The cost of treatment should be within reason for the type of service that is being provided.
4. Does the therapy promise to cure ASD or take the ASD away? What are the proposed benefits of participating in the therapy? What are treatment outcomes? Does the therapy make any promises, if so, what are the promises? Caution should be given to any treatment that promises to cure autism or promises absolutes in gains. Treatments should also have an evaluation component that can be explained to the participant.
5. Does the therapy seem like a good fit for the individual considering financial demands, time demands, and treatment expectations/processes?

Individuals should consider if the treatment approach is something they can commit their time, finances, and energy to before beginning.

6. How is the therapy governed or monitored? Participants should understand if there is any oversight for the treatment or the professional providing the treatment. If the therapy has no accountability this may be a caution for individuals regarding the treatment.

7. How is the professional implementing or selling the therapy considered a valid and reliable person to do so? Professionals or those implementing treatment should be able to communicate to families how they are qualified to implement the therapy.

Life with ASD

ASD does not have a singular look, feel, or experience. Just as the spectrum manifests many different "looks" of ASD, so life with autism can look many different ways depending on the individual and the impact their autism is having on their life. As Dr. Stephen Shore has famously coined "If you have met one child with autism, then you have met one child with autism." While acknowledging the individualized nature of autism, there are some commonalities for those living with an ASD.

A systemic issue – The myriad ways that autism can affect an individual weave throughout home life, extended family, school environment, community, and job environment. When working with autistic individuals it is critical to remember how encompassing the disorder is on the person's life. Everywhere the person goes, whether it be school, interacting with their family, going to work, or participating in a community event – their autism is present – it is not something that can be ignored or turned off for convenience.

School challenges – From the very beginnings of daycare and preschool and throughout college completion, individuals with autism face an uphill battle in most educational settings. The school setting can present some of the greatest challenges to an autistic person. The social and communication demands, processing requirements, and sensory experiences present in every school day can create great dysregulation for the person with autism. Many schools find themselves in inadequate positions to provide the level of services and resources that autistic individuals need to be their most successful. Professionals and parents can be beneficial in helping to educate school personnel about autism and providing suggestions for services and resources to facilitate a more successful learning experience.

A family with ASD – A diagnosis of autism affects the whole family. It is not unusual for the autistic individual to occupy most of the family's time, decisions, and resources. The Autism Society of America (2020) proposed that a child's autism diagnosis affects every member of the family in different ways. Parents must shift much of their resources of time and money towards providing treatment and interventions for their child, to the exclusion of other priorities. The needs of an autistic child complicate familial relationships, especially with siblings. However, parents can help their family by informing their other children about autism and the complications it introduces, understanding the challenges siblings face and helping them cope, and involving members of the extended family to create a network of help and understanding. Parents often must place their primary focus on helping their child with ASD, which can create a myriad of other concerns highlighted in Table 1.2.

Therapy and interventions – The intensity and duration of therapy and interventions that a person with ASD participates in will vary across the spectrum. It is likely that individuals with an autism diagnosis will participate in some form of therapy or intervention sometime during their lifetime. Some autistic individuals may consistently participate in therapies or interventions. Some individuals may enter and exit therapies and interventions as needed. Therapies and interventions may cover a whole variety of needs depending on the individual and the level of the individual's impairment, but common focus areas include social functioning, speech and language issues, independent living skills, emotional regulation ability, anxiety struggles, and executive functioning impairments. This could involve a child needing time off from school to attend a therapy session or an adult having a job coach present as they begin a new job. The basics of being autism friendly involves understanding and providing normality (instead of resistance) to the needs of those with ASD.

Self-acceptance – Autistic individuals will be in a continuous process of understanding themselves, their diagnosis and how it impacts the world around them, and how the world around them can create support or barriers. Gaining self-awareness of these issues will be critical for the individual with ASD to live their most independent life. Children around the late elementary and pre-teen years can begin to learn more about their diagnosis and how it impacts them. As they grow and mature, they should

Table 1.2 Typical Family Stressors Associated with ASD

Extra stress on the marriage relationship
Sibling issues including feeling neglected, feeling angry, and taking on a parenting role
A strain on finances, especially regarding the cost of therapies
Extra time off from work for appointments and crisis intervention
A strain in external family relationships
Isolation in social and community involvement
Difficulty obtaining respite and self-care
Education challenges

master self-advocacy skills and become the best expert on themselves and their diagnosis. Those involved with individuals with autism are instrumental in how the autistic person gains self-acceptance skills by how they treat, value, and respond to those with ASD.

Educating others – Individuals with autism will find much of their time spent educating others about ASD, specifically how their own ASD manifests and impacts them. Although education and awareness initiatives continue to increase, there still exists much inaccurate information, ignorance, and stereotyping regarding autism. Unfortunately, some autistic individuals have found it easier to not disclose they have autism because of the mislabeling and stigmatization that can occur. Inevitably, those with an ASD diagnosis will find themselves in situations where it will be necessary to educate those around them about autism. The autism friendly professional listens to those with ASD, is willing to learn, and above all else values the totality of the autistic person.

The world of autism is a vast and often a complex place with many variables, thoughts, and opinions. Autistic individuals must learn to understand themselves and how their unique person maneuvers in the greater world in which they live. Just as the individual with autism is on a journey, those who work with, interact, educate, serve, and help those with ASD are also on a journey. Their journey involves increasing their willingness to understand and increase awareness of the autistic individual. Their process of becoming autism friendly means being caring, kind, and making the effort to value differences and see the strengths that the autistic person brings to any setting. For the autism friendly professional, it is not just learning about autism but applying that knowledge to the real people they encounter each day.

2 How Autism Affects Children

Autism can affect children in a myriad of different ways. One of the challenges for the lay professional is understanding the various ways ASD can manifest. Autistic children may have some similar unifying presentations, but the severity of their needs and the presence or absence of other features will vary, such as fine motor ability, intelligence, increased or decreased verbal output, and social strengths (Coplan, 2010). Autism is a spectrum disorder, meaning there are many manifestations and ways a child or adolescent could be affected. Siri and Lyons (2010) suggested that ASD is difficult to define; no two children have the same set of symptoms. Each child may broadly share common general manifestations but the triggers and causes for these manifestations may vary greatly from one child to another.

Howard et al. (2017) stated that children with ASD typically show needs in early infancy, namely in the areas of play, stereotypical behaviors, and shared attention. They tend to struggle with symbolic play and prefer to play alone, and they show a preference for toys based on sensory stimulation. Autistic children may display a repetitive and stereotypical quality to their play and it can be challenging for peers to navigate when they are trying to engage with the child with ASD. Further, challenges with perspective taking may contribute to social struggles which impede successful peer interactions. This becomes important awareness for schools, after school programs, daycares, summer camps, and other environments where play and social skills are primary.

Wolfberg (1999) proposed that children must be able to enter a social group and coordinate the mutual activity to engage in play with peers or other partners. Play supports the exploration of social roles when children learn to negotiate, compromise, and become aware of and understand the mental states of others. Autistic children who lack play skills, specifically in the areas of pretend, symbolic, and peer play, are highly susceptible to being left out and rejected by neurotypical peers. They are susceptible to being socially isolated, bullied, and developing a negative self-worth. Further, they miss out not only on peer social benefits of play but a whole host of other learning and problem-solving mechanisms that are typically developed through play.

DOI: 10.4324/9781003105633-3

Koenig (2012) asserted that children and adolescents with ASD have neurobiological differences that make them less predisposed to engage in social interaction. Throughout development, autistic children are less responsive to the social environment in general and do not benefit from the many implicit social learning experiences available from day-to-day experiences. Syriopoulou-Delli et al. (2018) stated that one of the core symptoms of ASD is a difference in social functioning. Differences include difficulties in initiating or joining social activities, difficulties in understanding others' viewpoints, engaging in inappropriate behaviors, lack of eye contact, distance from people, non-functional use of language, and a lack of communicative gestures.

The term "social skill" covers a wide range and variety of skills from simple to complex (Grant & Turner-Bumberry, 2020). Social skills can be anything from learning to take turns, to knowing when a situation is unsafe, to giving a public speech. Social skills are interpersonal, specific behaviors that permit an individual to interact successfully with others in the environment. The extent to which an individual is considered to have adequate social skills is determined by others. This is especially true for children and adolescents with autism, as they may not be able to fully understand or recognize a social skill even after they have obtained it (Grant 2017a). Many autistic children will struggle on some level with social functioning/navigation and each child will possess social strengths. The autism friendly professional should support growth in social skill needs while simultaneously recognizing and encouraging social strengths.

A need in social navigation is a common symptom among all those with ASD. It is highly likely that any child diagnosed with autism will need help in learning social skills. The negative outcomes associated with a lack of social skills can be many and serious. The inability to understand social functioning and possess social skills can create high levels of anxiety in children with autism and create problems in school and community settings. Research has shown that these difficulties with social functioning are present even for the most cognitively able individuals on the spectrum (Reichow & Volkmar, 2010).

Early on, autistic children demonstrate social skill processes that differentiate them from their typical peers and classmates. In elementary school, they might have important relational problems such as difficulties initiating and maintaining friendships with others (Kasari et al, 2016; Reichow & Volkmar, 2010). In high school, individuals with ASD might continue to show evidence of the same difficulties experienced in childhood, placing them at risk for rejection and victimization by their peer group. These problems could ultimately lead to social isolation, psychopathology, and poor academic achievement. Research also contends that autistic individuals do not simply outgrow their social skills challenges; rather these difficulties might persist into their adult life and could continue to negatively affect their social functioning (D'Amico & Lalonde, 2017).

When working with autistic children and adolescents, it is critical for professionals to assess and conceptualize each individual child with autism to fully understand how the ASD manifests for the particular child. Although there may be some commonalities, each child with ASD will present with their unique struggles, needs, and strengths. Professionals who work with autistic children are encouraged to develop a formal assessment procedure to help the professional more accurately identify each child's skill strengths and skill needs as well as any particulars a child might be experiencing due to other issues. This process can be accomplished through parent-completed inventories, professional observations, and simply spending time with the child and obtaining background information from the child's parents.

Anastasia Phelps, *My Life with Autism*

Anastasia Phelps is a 17-year-old spoken word artist with autism. Among her many activities, she dedicates herself to advocating for those who are differently abled through public speaking, writing, and expressive arts. In her writing (*My Life with Autism*) she shares her perspective and experiences about being a child with autism. More about Anastasia can be found on her Beautiful Not Broken Facebook page.

> Unhealthy comparison has always been an issue of mine. The best example I can think of was when I was in the second grade. I often went out into the playground and sat with my notebook and markers; scribbling away while the other kids played. My hand only broke its rhythm when my eyes strayed, with much longing, over to my joyfully playing peers.
>
> Over the past 17 years, I felt like an inadequate weirdo who was always striving too far, only to never get anywhere. On top of that, my medications always seemed to complicate my emotions and play with my perception, which really didn't help me much.
>
> Over the years, I had developed such harsh views of myself. Not only that . . . I have also become so attached to the thoughts and opinions of others. It is a very unhealthy addiction for me – about as harmful to my mind as excessive amounts of drugs or alcohol might be to any individual.
>
> It is hard when all I can see is my autism . . . but, even harder than that, is when all anyone else seems to see in me is my autism. I do not possess telepathic abilities . . . I cannot tell what you see in me. I can only take a guess. So, I like it when people talk to me like I am another human being like anyone else. I like it when they give me a chance instead of writing me off as a weirdo.
>
> Just like anyone else, I want acceptance, and I want to be listened to.

I have had quite a few people talk to me like I am an infant. I have had former therapists address me in such tones, and even leaders and students from my church would talk to me in the same demeaning manner. The thing is, I know 90% of them don't necessarily do it with bad intent, however, that doesn't make it any less discouraging or hurtful to me.

I have a really hard time properly reacting to someone's emotions in the moment, but it doesn't mean I cannot feel for them or care. I just have a really hard time expressing my thoughts and feelings. It is almost like I am disconnected, and my thoughts and actions run off in opposite directions. It can be so frustrating at times.

Whether we are verbal or nonverbal, advocacy is a real struggle for those on the autism spectrum. Even as an autism advocate, I find it hard in my everyday life, to communicate my thoughts and feelings in an efficient manner.

Something my mother and I have learned throughout the years is that advocacy is a never-ending journey for both the parent and the child.

It is exceedingly difficult, even near impossible for those of us on spectrum to build that bridge, between where we are and where we are expected to be. For example, it is already enough of a stretch to expect a "neurotypical" teen or child to be aware of what they need, let alone express exactly what it is. So why would you expect someone who has difficulty communicating, to be able to advocate for themselves in a way that you will understand?

If the child doesn't give you clear answers, it doesn't necessarily mean they don't have more to say. Most likely than not, they are uncomfortable. So much more goes on underneath the surface, beneath what can be seen with eyes alone. Everyone deserves an advocate; everyone deserves to be heard.

As a teen, I still struggle to insert myself in group conversations. I struggle to find openings where I can talk and yet not interrupt the others who wish to speak, or who may not have been finished. It really throws my mind into a frenzy.

Oftentimes, especially among my peers, I just don't know how to express myself. I am conflicted on how to react socially, so I tend to watch rather than interact. Which sometimes results in me being perceived as stuck up or outlandish. The thing is, I can keep up with the conversation mentally, and as long as it is a topic I am familiar with, I can even join in. But I would rather not risk embarrassing myself socially if I can help it, since I already feel like everyone is already judging me.

The most important thing I want people to see, is that I am not autism, and autism is not me. It is a source of some of my weaknesses and some of my strengths - nothing more, nothing less. Just like you have your weaknesses and strengths, I have mine.

And though autism is a foundation, it is not the entire structure of who I am; though autism is one piece of my mental puzzle, it is not the entire picture.

I want people to remember that.

Common Struggle Areas

A child or adolescent with ASD will almost always need an individual assessment to accurately identify their struggle areas, skills strengths, and preferences. Although it is understood that each child will have their unique manifestation regarding their ASD, there are some common need areas that tend to affect most children with autism at varying levels.

Communication skills – Children with ASD will vary in their communication strengths and needs. Most children with autism will have some level of communication challenge. Some children will present as nonverbal. Other children may possess a large vocabulary but lack ability to connect words verbally to their emotions or may lack in being able to participate in reciprocal conversation.

Writing skills – Autistic children tend to have an aversion to writing, they may prefer to listen to, watch, or do instead of writing (Attwood & Garnett, 2013). Many children with ASD prefer using a keyboard and seem to be more successful when allowed to do so. Writing should be approached with an awareness that children with autism will need specific and realistic expectations and support.

Receptive language – Children with ASD may have receptive language challenges. Many of these children may display average or above average ability in expressive language. There can be a large discrepancy between receptive and expressive language ability. Receptive language refers to the child's ability to take in or receive language. A child with receptive language needs will likely not hear or process important pieces of information that are being communicated to them verbally.

Play skills – Autistic children usually do not display pretend or imaginary play and peer or group play. Regarding peer or group play, children with ASD typically do desire to participate and interact with other peers in group play but lack the skills to interact successfully and find the experience to be too overwhelming. Thus, most attempts at peer interaction, especially with neurotypical peers, are not successful and may even create additional issues. Regarding pretend and imaginative play, children with autism may lack the neurological process of understanding pretend, symbolism, and metaphor (Grant 2017b).

Generalization ability – Many children with ASD will struggle with generalizing information. A child may learn a social skill in one context and have a difficult time generalizing the same basic skill to another context.

There may be struggles with understanding nuance, learning through concepts, generalities, subjective situations, and pulling from an existing knowledge base to apply to new or unfamiliar scenarios. This is an important consideration when working with and serving children with ASD.

Rigid (literal) thinking – Autistic children may think in a rigid way. This means they may be very literal in their thinking, struggle with abstract concepts, prefer more concrete thoughts, and find it difficult to consider alternatives or to accept when things are not how they expected or believed they should be. It can be difficult for children to think ahead and to guess what is going to happen next, which means that they may become anxious or confused in some situations, especially new situations. Professionals can assist children by establishing consistent and predictable routines while systematically introducing coping skills designed to help children process changes and manage unpredictable situations.

Processing speed – Research has shown children with ASD were found to have selective needs in executive function. Executive dysfunction regarding attention, set shifting, planning, and processing speed have been reported in young autistic children. Regarding executive function struggles, processing speed was found to be one of the weakest areas for autistic children. Processing speed deficits present significant challenges for children in educational settings, home settings, and any setting where they are required to take in information and perform task completion.

Fear of making mistakes – Children with ASD are prone to developing an almost pathological fear of failure, errors, or making a mistake. This fear may cause children to be resistant to trying new experiences or participating in programs. Professionals will want to reinforce a child's abilities and encourage self-confidence (Attwood & Garnett, 2013).

Regulation ability – A need in social skills, play skills, ability to regulate emotions, and sensory processing challenges can all manifest a great deal of unrest and unwanted behavioral presentation for the autistic child (Grant, 2017a). This behavior manifestation is typically the result of the child or adolescent becoming too dysregulated. Most children with autism will lack the ability to recognize when they are becoming dysregulated, lack the ability to regulate their system, and lack coping skills to implement when they are becoming dysregulated. Often, dysregulation behaviors can be misinterpreted as oppositional or defiant behaviors.

Social functioning – Autistic children typically do desire to have friendships and interact with other peers, but simply lack the social ability and skills to interact successfully. Thus, most attempts at some type of interaction are met with rejection and anxiety for the child with autism. Repeated attempts to engage socially, without possessing the appropriate social skills, can create a host of other issues including strong poor self-worth and negative cognitions that are difficult to regulate (Grant 2017a). Social function needs are arguably the most common issue with children diagnosed with ASD regardless of where the child may be on the spectrum. Certainly, the level of social functioning need will vary but each child with ASD will manifest with some level of social challenge.

Education struggles – Arguably the most challenging environment for autistic children is a school setting. The sensory input, social navigation, academic challenges, randomness, constantly changing (unexpected) nature of a typical school creates an almost anti-environment for a child with ASD. Many autistic children struggle navigating a school day with little support to help them be successful.

Sensory input issues – A common manifestation in children with ASD is experiencing sensory processing challenges. These challenges can be in one or more of the eight sensory areas and basically involve a sensory processing "traffic jam" in the brain where sensory input cannot be appropriately modulated. Sensory challenges can be difficult to identify, diagnose, and understand. Often, the lay professional does not see or understand the sensory challenges the child with autism is facing. These challenges can produce a host of unwanted behaviors including avoidance, opposition, eloping, and meltdown.

Public events – Autistic children typically have a threshold of how much social, sensory, and other stimulation they can manage in any given day/week. Going out in public to a grocery store, a school play, an outdoor city event, etc. can be problematic if the child with ASD is not properly regulated or has already been experiencing many of these events. Often autistic children need a mindful approach to how much challenge and stimulation is being presented for them on a daily basis with extra care given to make sure they have down, relaxing, and regulating time in their schedule.

Being consistent with behavior – Autistic children often have splintered skill development meaning they may be able to do something very well and struggle to do a similar skill. Their behavior is often inconsistent and not predictable. This is due to their development and regulation struggles. A child with ASD may do well on something one day and struggle with something else the next day which seems easier and more doable.

Self-reflection (introspection) – Self-reflection is processed differently by the brains of children with ASD. Some autistic children may lack an inner voice or introspective ability and think in pictures rather than words. There is a challenge for these children to look within themselves and process strengths and weaknesses and formulate a change/growth plan. Children who may possess some introspection ability, will still have difficulty translating their visual thoughts into words. Professionals can help children gain self-reflective ability by utilizing visual learning tools to teach introspective concepts.

Self-advocacy – Milestones Autism Resources (2020) described self-advocacy as an individual's ability to effectively communicate, convey, negotiate, or assert their own interests, desires, needs, and rights. It involves making informed decisions and taking responsibility for those decisions. Self-knowledge is the first step towards self-advocacy. An autistic child must know their strengths, needs, and interests before they can begin to advocate. Self-advocacy skills should be learned as early as possible and begin by learning how to make personal choices, such as making choices about what to eat, how to spend one's free time, and what to do after graduating from high school. The Milestones Autism website (www.milestones.org) lists several self-advocacy skills by age that children and adolescents with ASD should strive to accomplish.

Autistic children cannot possibly be conceptualized into one manifestation. The variance of presentation and effect of the autism is large. It has often been said if there are 100 children in the next room with autism, then you have 100 different "looks" of autism in the next room. Grant (2017a) reported that although children with ASD vary considerably in terms of their ASD affect, they may present in certain ways and struggle with particular constructs that should be noted.

- It is possible autistic children will have social skill needs and high levels of discomfort in social situations regardless of their level of social functioning. Social situations, even those that may seem benign to neurotypical individuals may be very stress producing and challenging to children with ASD. Children with autism may resist, refuse, elope, or become oppositional when asked to participate in anxiety producing social situations.
- Autistic children may poorly modulate their emotions (identifying and expressing emotions). Children with ASD may not understand what emotions are and cannot identify what they are feeling or how to express a feeling in an appropriate manner. Emotions may manifest as unwanted behaviors – behavior is typically communicating a feeling or need.
- For autistic children there can be struggles with anxiety and high levels of dysregulation. Anxiety is typically the most challenging negative emotion for a child with ASD. Anxiety can look like avoidance, withdrawn behavior, refusing to cooperate, and even large meltdowns.
- Autistic children may be experiencing some level of dysregulation; the question is how much? Many things can create dysregulation including poor regulation ability, a lack of social skills, new or unexpected situations, and sensory issues. The inability to regulate their system can lead to unwanted behaviors that can be misunderstood as oppositional defiant behavior or planned behavior when it is typically an uncontrollable state.
- It is likely children with ASD will produce most unwanted behavior episodes out of a result of being dysregulated, which is typically not

premeditated or controlled by the child and is often a very frightening experience for the child. This is an extremely fearful state for the child who often does not understand what is happening to their system or how to gain control.

- Autistic children may have problems handling transitions, changes to their schedule or routine, and new people or experiences. Any spontaneous happening will likely produce anxiety and discomfort. Children with autism will manage better with a known schedule including transitions. Spontaneous occurrences often create dysregulation.
- Often, autistic children appear more capable or less capable than their cognitive level. Children with a less impaired manifestation can often "pass" as neurotypical and others may not understand they have challenges. This can lead to unrealistic expectations that the child cannot reach and less patience on the part of the professional. Conversely, some children may appear more impaired and professionals may lower their expectations and treat the child in rudimentary ways which are beneath their cognitive and skill ability.
- Autistic children may have small and large motor and coordination challenges. It is common for children with ASD to struggle with motor skills which may limit what they can do in small and large motor movement activities.
- Usually children with ASD are experiencing a great many sensory processing issues in one or multiple areas regarding the eight senses. Sensory struggles can be challenging to identify and may involve environmental issues that seem benign to the professional. Sensory struggles are another area that can create dysregulation for the child.
- It is likely children with autism are a visual learner and prefer information presented in a visual format. Autistic children are often strong visual learners. Information presented verbally without a visual component is less likely to be processed, retained, and recalled by the child with autism.
- Typically, autistic children are concrete and literal thinkers. They will likely not do well with abstract or subjective thoughts and processes or information presented in this format. Children with ASD often think literally not figuratively. They prefer information and conversation that is concrete and not presented in analogy or metaphor. The latter can create confusion and misunderstanding for the child.
- Children with autism may struggle verbally to communicate what they are thinking or feeling especially when they are in a dysregulated state. Communication skills (verbal and nonverbal) may not be strong skills in children with ASD. It is also well known that the more dysregulated an autistic child becomes, the less they communicate verbally.
- Autistic children usually have challenges in receptive language ability even when their expressive language ability is high. Some children with ASD can speak like adults and present information verbally at

an advanced level. This often does not match how they take in verbal information (receptive language). These differences can create missed information and lack of follow-through on tasks and work especially when the information is presented to the child in exclusively verbal format.

- Likely children with ASD will be inconsistent in terms of skill presentation. They may accomplish something one day that seems very challenging and the next day they are unable to accomplish something that seems much less difficult. Professionals will observe splintered skill development and uneven skill development that does not always progress in a linear fashion.
- Autistic children may present with a great deal of hyperarousal (over-responsiveness to stimuli and one's environment, for example jumpy, finding it hard to concentrate, and being impulsive) or be the exact opposite and present with a great deal of hypoarousal (under-responsiveness to stimuli and one's environment, for example, as lethargy, inattention, apathy, or boredom).
- For autistic children there is a susceptibility to being bullied at school and in peer situations. This often occurs in school settings or group peer situations. Often autistic children (especially those with fewer impairments) are easy targets for bullies and they may not understand what is occurring or how to respond/react.
- Children with ASD may pause to respond to questions or tasks. They may need extra time to process what has been said or asked of them. Slower processing speed is one of the more researched differences in those with ASD. This may appear as the child taking longer to respond to questions or longer to answer. The child is processing and can respond but may need additional time.
- It is likely autistic children will experience school as the most demanding and dysregulating environment in which they participate. Schools present the antithesis to children with ASD resulting in many children disliking school and resisting going to school. There exists a myriad of issues and struggles and much advocacy work is done to help children with autism be successful in school settings.

Supporting Children with ASD

Professionals across multiple settings have the opportunity to support autistic children. Many autistic children find themselves on the opposite end from support. Many are criticized, misunderstood, and treated badly by others. As professionals increase their awareness and understanding of ASD, they are positioned to come alongside autistic children and offer support, encouragement, and validation.

There are multiple ways professionals can support children with autism. Support begins with becoming educated and learning about autism, how it affects children, and the personal experiences of children and families affected by autism. Supporting autistic children means supporting parents. Support involves avoiding judgment of parents and instead aiding, asking how help can be provided, and offering to listen to their needs and struggles. A sincere attempt to help and provide support can make a successful difference for an autistic child. Some additional ways to support children with autism include:

- get to know the child beyond the ASD. Develop a relationship with the child,
- find out what the child likes, what their interests are, and what they enjoy,
- focus on the child's strengths, what they do well, and recognize their accomplishments,
- avoid focusing on the child's negative behavior and make everything about their behavior,
- keep an open mind to continue to learn about autism,
- remember the autistic child may have a different learning style,
- remember the child with ASD may need a different environmental set up,
- think about keeping the environment sensory friendly, minimizing distractions, and keeping things organized,
- allow autistic children to have a favorite item or toy that may be regulating or soothing for them,
- and be patient and not taking behaviors personally.

Recognizing Strengths in Children with ASD

Recognizing strengths in autistic children and valuing neurodiversity has significant benefits. It can help children (and their parents) frame their challenges as differences, rather than deficits. It can also shed light on instructional approaches that might help to highlight particular strengths. It also normalizes the fact that there are many productive individual members of society who are not neurotypical and different ways of thinking, processing, and responding can be valuable. When neurotypical individuals understand neurodiversity, children with autism are more accepted and appreciated in the social settings and situations where they may already be facing certain challenges.

It is important to focus on the positives when discussing children on the spectrum with other neurotypical children and adults. Talking about an autistic child's skills and successes is crucial to teaching other children and adults to view ASD through a more positive lens. It is also important to incorporate the child on the spectrum in the conversation, allowing them to express what they feel when they experience sensory challenges, dysregulation, or display awkward social behavior. Neurodiversity initiatives mean explaining to others that autistic children process information a little

Table 2.1 Typical Strengths Found in Children with Autism

Honest and trustworthy

Visual learner

Follows rules

Advanced knowledge in special topics of interest

Rote memory skills

Provide a different perspective

No hidden intentions or passive aggressive behaviors

Loyal to people and processes

differently and that can change the way they communicate in social situations and how they express when they feel uncomfortable or overwhelmed. Luck & Barboa (2015) created the *Albert* book series which focuses on a young child and his experience with autism. Books such as these can be a valuable tool in helping other children gain better positive awareness of autism.

Often children with ASD are seen as having a diagnosis which usually carries a host of stigmas and negative assumptions about how the child is going to present. This view diminishes and hides any recognition of the child's strengths. It creates a situation which makes the child a behavior (usually negative behavior) instead of a fully functioning unique individual with a host of abilities and strengths despite their challenges. Table 2.1 highlights some of the strengths that can be recognized about autistic children.

Johnny's Story

Background – Johnny was diagnosed with ASD at age four. Prior to his ASD diagnosis, Johnny was diagnosed with a chromosome disorder and intellectual development disorder (IDD). Besides his developmental issues, Johnny experienced a large number of medically related problems. He lived with his mother and father and an older brother who was also diagnosed with autism but had fewer impairments than Johnny. In his preschool years, Johnny stayed at home with his mother mostly due to daycare and preschool not being able to work with Johnny. When he was old enough, he began kindergarten and had an incredibly challenging year in the public school he attended. The school was poorly equipped and trained to help Johnny with the issues in which he struggled. He was mostly nonverbal, with little attunement ability. Most of Johnny's kindergarten year was spent sitting in a corner with whatever toy or material would occupy him. He did have an IEP but his goals and implementation of any plan rarely materialized.

Toward the end of his kindergarten year, Johnny's mother realized the school could not help her child. She petitioned to have him placed in a state school for children with more severe impairments. This request was approved, and Johnny spent most of his education in the state school advancing in academic and functional skills. Through his childhood years, Johnny was able to advance in his verbal and attunement ability. He also made advances in being able to do several things independently, but by age 18, he could not function on his own or make important decisions without assistance. His parents acquired guardianship of Johnny and he began an adult school program focused on teaching independent living skills. His parents also acquired an in-home assist through the Department of Mental Health to aid in furthering Johnny's skill development.

Throughout Johnny's childhood, he and his family experienced many difficulties. The educational challenges were consistent. He also consistently experienced medical issues and had to be hospitalized multiple times and was involved with several specialists. Johnny's parents were very insightful and proactive about supporting Johnny and acquiring any needed services. They were active in advocating for him and focused on moving him forward in skill development. There were regular family stressors due to Johnny's conditions, but his family support was strong.

Struggle areas – A primary struggle area in Johnny's childhood was education/academic issues. There was quite an extensive process to get an appropriate educational environment established for Johnny. Often the school setting was not accommodating and not supportive. Most of Johnny's educational success was due to his parent's strong advocacy skills. Johnny also experienced a high level of anxiety. At times, his anxiety levels were debilitating. Johnny struggled with anxiety throughout the majority of this childhood. He had difficulty learning potty training and this was an ongoing issue throughout childhood and into adult life. Johnny's cognitive development was low and remained low throughout his childhood, which created multiple struggles for Johnny, including learning new skills and advancing in education and functional ability. He was also affected by poor fine and large motor skills which, at times, required that he use a wheelchair. Lastly, Johnny struggled with being able to do many things independently. Although he did gain skills, many areas in his life required assistance.

Strengths – Johnny was a very social child, he enjoyed being around other people and interacting with other people, Johnny's parents were very diligent about involving Johnny in social activities and being consistent in this throughout his childhood. Johnny also enjoyed playing independently and with others. He would freely engage in play if given the opportunity. Although Johnny had limits in verbal ability and social skills, he was as active as he could be in socialization and play.

He was very drawn to and capable with electronics. He was able to understand and manipulate video games and apps almost without deficit.

He seemed to have a special knowledge ability when participating with electronics. Johnny could easily form special interests in certain topics and become very experienced and familiar with the topic. This gave him a knowledge ability in a specific area that was equal or above his peers. Johnny was a very cooperative child. He would easily participate (at his ability level) and was open to others giving him instruction and working with him on task completion.

Supports and services – Throughout Johnny's childhood, he received multiple services and supports. He had an IEP and received special services at school and attended a state school for children with developmental issues. He received multiple in-home support services from in-home specialists. He received speech therapy, occupational therapy, and Aut-Play® Therapy (a specialized form of play therapy designed for autistic children). He also regularly saw a neurologist and several other medical professionals. Johnny also received a great deal of support from his family, his church, family friends, and the community in which he lived.

Autism friendly experience – Johnny's autism friendly experience can best be described as a combination of positive and negative. On the positive side, Johnny received a great deal of care and value from his family, family friends, and individuals in his community. He also experienced very caring and attentive professionals who worked with him and his family. On the negative side, the school system often devalued and neglected him and was often judgmental toward his parents. There were multiple instances in the community where Johnny was dismissed as a lost cause and treated poorly. This happened in church settings, in hospital settings, and with extended family members. Through the diligence of his parents, eventually Johnny had a strong support system of family, community, and professionals but it did not materialize early or without his parent's advocacy and persistence.

Kenzie's Story

Background – Kenzie was diagnosed with ASD at age five. Her manifestation with autism was a mild impairment and included some sensory issues and regulation challenges. Her official diagnosis at the time was Asperger's syndrome. Later in childhood she would score as gifted academically and be diagnosed with Pediatric Autoimmune Neuropsychiatric Disorders Associated with Streptococcal Infections (PANDAS). She lived with her mother and one younger brother and older sister (both neurotypical).

Kenzie began public school in kindergarten and remained in public school until second grade. Her first two years of school were extremely challenging. She was given an IEP and provided some special accommodations, but she struggled to get through school days. She had many challenges with the social aspects of school and would often become dysregulated and have large meltdowns at school which would result in her mother being contacted to come and get her from school. The school had difficulty understanding Kenzie's regulation challenges and would regularly threaten to expel her from school if there continued to be behavior problems.

Kenzie's mother removed her from the public school after her first-grade year and began homeschooling. Kenzie's behaviors improved but she continued to have some meltdowns at home especially when she was challenged with new people or situations. Her academic performance improved greatly being homeschooled and she advanced in areas beyond her grade level. The summer before her fifth-grade year, Kenzie decided she would like to try formal school again and had the opportunity to attend a private school focused on working with autistic children. The beginning of the private school experience was challenging, mainly due to social struggles and anxiety. The school worked well with Kenzie to help her adjust to social situations and provided regulating experiences for her. By the end of her fifth-grade year, she was thriving in the social environment at school. She also continued to advance academically, being able to participate in a gifted classroom. She was able to stabilize socially and academically remaining in the private school until she graduated high school.

Throughout Kenzie's childhood, she struggled with social skills. Any social situation would often create high levels of anxiety and confusion which would lead to a dysregulated state which almost always turned into a behavior meltdown. Because Kenzie appeared neurotypical to the casual observer, she was often mislabeled, misunderstood, and challenged/ addressed in ways that she could not understand. Kenzie's mother spent a great deal of time advocating and explaining for her daughter and trying to teach Kenzie to advocate for herself. In friend settings, church settings, extracurricular settings, and various other public/social situations, Kenzie would struggle, be judged, and feel rejected. This was a hallmark of Kenzie's childhood experiences up until she reached sixth grade when due to proper interventions, Kenzie's skill deficits improved.

Struggle areas – Kenzie struggled with educational services up to her middle school years. She had difficulties with the overwhelming environment of public school and the school system did not understand Kenzie's issues and provided little support for her. One of Kenzie's most challenging struggles involved social functioning. Kenzie lacked social skills, found social situations confusing, and typically experienced anxiety going into and participating in social situations. Medically, she struggled with her PANDAS diagnosis. It was a process for her family and herself to understand the diagnosis and how it affected her. It was also a process to find professionals to work with her in treating the condition.

Strengths – Kenzie was a gifted child; her academic ability was a high strength for her. She could achieve academically well beyond her peers. She also possessed high cognitive ability and when she was regulated, could process very effectively. She had advanced expressive language and reading ability which helped her with academic success and advocacy skills. Kenzie's personality was very engaging; she was a well-spoken and engaging child. Many adults responded well to Kenzie if she was not in a dysregulated condition. She also possessed advanced advocacy skills during her childhood. She was often able to advocate effectively for her needs.

Supports and services – Kenzie had a great deal of support from her immediate and extended family. Along with her mother, she was valued and understood by her grandparents and other extended family members. Kenzie also found support in the private autism school she began in fifth grade. This proved to be a significant experience for her, to be in an educational environment that did not mislabel her and strived to encourage and help her. She also participated in occupational therapy, AutPlay® Therapy, and occasionally had medication support.

Autism friendly experience – Kenzie's autism friendly experience would best be described as a roller coaster of misunderstanding, mislabeling, and rejection. Outside of Kenzie's family members, most of her experience with others was met with mislabeling her as a problem child, disrespectful, or a "brat." Kenzie would understand this rejection, which led to more social anxiety problems. Eventually Kenzie's mother found supportive professionals to work with Kenzie and by middle school was in a supportive educational setting. It took Kenzie a lot of interventions and years to overcome the social stigma trauma she experienced being rejected in so many situations. Being able to eventually find autism friendly supports outside of her family members helped Kenzie overcome her social anxiety and negative past encounters and develop a positive social experience.

Autistic children are arguably one of our most vulnerable populations. They live with a way of processing and responding that is not mainstream accepted culture, not valued, and often misunderstood. They try to navigate a world with limited communication ability and developmental delays which so often lead to a confusing and scary navigation. If children with ASD are to be successful and live their best life, reaching their fullest potential, it must be with the assistance and guidance of caring, knowledgeable, and friendly adults who are willing to merge the waters of neurodiversity acceptance with empowering skill development. The autism friendly professional is never more needed than in the lives of autistic children and the positive and long-term impact of their presence cannot be underestimated. These early years set the foundation and course for becoming an accomplished autistic adult. The influence that the adult professional (across settings) has on children with autism is immeasurable. They have the ability to move the child forward or set them back. This makes becoming an autism friendly professional so vital to the success of autistic children.

3 How Autism Affects Adults

A study from the Centers for Disease Control and Prevention (CDC) (2020) estimated the prevalence of autism spectrum disorder (ASD) among adults aged 18 years and older in the United States to be 5,437,988 or (2.21%). The prevalence of US adults with ASD ranged from a low of 1.97% in Louisiana to a high of 2.42% in Massachusetts. The states with the greatest estimated number of adults living with ASD included California (701,669), Texas (449,631), New York (342,280), and Florida (329,131). Consistent with estimates of ASD in US school-aged children, prevalence was found to be higher in men than in women.

Over the last few years more and more autistic adults have been writing about, speaking about, and training others about their experiences living with ASD. The skills they share about surviving in the neurotypical world provide ideas and awareness to others with ASD and those who work with and serve autistic individuals. Sicile-Kira (2004) stated that more is known about autistic adults than ever before. Many autistic adults have written personal accounts of what their lives are like, and how they have overcome challenges to make living in a neurotypical world easier. Their insights have been powerful in providing new ideas about living, socializing, and work strategies and successes for those with autism.

The life of an autistic adult often involves quite different implications from childhood. Some adults with ASD can live independently with no assistance from another person. They are able to navigate their personal and work life much in the same way a neurotypical individual would and are able to manage any ASD related issues that materialize. Other autistic adults may need some type of support to effectively navigate their adult life. This support may be minimal in the way of a job coach, or attending a specific therapy, or some type of assisted living experience. Some autistic adults may require consistent support and need help with basic life functioning and are unable to live independently or make decisions on their own. The same variance across the spectrum of autism which exists for children also exists for adults with ASD.

Living with autism can be conceptualized as a process – transitioning to adulthood is a process, and the process continues throughout adulthood.

DOI: 10.4324/9781003105633-4

The transition begins the day the child is born. Steps along the way include the first time the child is left with a sitter, the first time they are sent to spend the night with a grandparent, or the first time they go to camp or school. For an individual with ASD, steps in transition to adulthood may include in home or out of home respite care, a trial stay at a group home, the first attempt at a part-time job, volunteering, or working in a supported employment setting. Each of these moments entails a piece of independence and mastery. They become essential parts of the process of becoming a competent adult and define the adult experience for the autistic individual (Coplan, 2010).

It would be impossible to capture a single or even a few descriptors of autism in adults and assume that would cover what ASD in adults looks like. Even though there are often similarities in experience and overlapping struggle areas, the variance of manifestation and affect is massive. For the purpose of better understanding and becoming more autism friendly, a variety of vignettes (autism "looks") are presented:

- Post high school may involve attending college for those with autism. Some autistic adults may attend and complete college without accessing resources or accommodations, others may be formally connected with college resources or have outside help with tutoring, communication, and time management skills.
- Some autistic adults are happily married and parenting children. Others may be single and have struggled to connect and get into a relationship. Others may be married but are struggling in their marriage and in parenting their children.
- Living at home with parents or other family members who are the primary caretakers may be the situation for some adults with ASD. They may not have the ability or independence skills to live on their own.
- Some adults may be living in an assisted living facility or apartment complex receiving some level of assistance with life management. The assistance can vary greatly based on the need. Some adults may be living in a fully monitored group facility where the state or governing agency has legal guardianship.
- Autistic adults may be living successfully on their own, renting or owning their own home without complication.
- Some adults may be receiving disability services benefits, and some may be accessing health insurance through their employer and others may have no health coverage.
- Adults with autism might be working in a fulltime job or working part time depending on their ability and desire. Some may be doing well in their work life while others are struggling with work social environments and methods of communication. Others may be struggling to find employment and utilizing the services of a job coach/program while others may not be able to work.

- Some autistic adults are vocal and successful advocates for those with ASD. They regularly speak, write, and train about their experiences with autism and how to help others with autism.
- Some autistic adults purposefully choose to maintain anonymity regarding having autism and others would not know they have the diagnosis.
- Some adults are unable to work or live independently due to their impairments. Their parents have guardianship, take care of them, and make most decisions for them. Some are working full time, living in their own home, and attending a post college specialty program. They can live independently but struggle with social situations and relationships.
- Many of these "looks" can overlap and combine, such as an autistic adult might be attending college without accommodations but needs to live with their parents due to deficits in independent living skills. Essentially hundreds of vignette examples could be created to illustrate the diversity of the autistic adult. Table 3.1 highlights Rodden's (2020) typical presentations of ASD in adults at home and at work.

One of the most debilitating ways in which autism can affect adults is the area of stigmatization. Gates (2019) defined stigma as targeting people on the basis of beliefs about them that have nothing to do with who they are. It undermines a person's humanity and overshadows the fullness of their identity by placing assumptions about negatively perceived qualities over openness to their actual personhood. For many autistic adults stigma experiences can lead to low self-worth, depression, and trauma responses. Botha & Frost (2019) found that social stress related to the stigma experienced by those with autism was predictive of higher levels of psychological distress and lower levels of emotional, psychological, and social well-being. Importantly, the research showed that these unique forms of minority stress could explain the mental health problems of autistic people above and beyond the effects of general and everyday forms of stress not related to stigma.

Stigma can manifest many ways for autistic adults and typically begins in childhood. Stigma can be thought of as a form of ableism which is defined as the discrimination of and social prejudice against people with disabilities or who are differently abled based on the belief that typical abilities are superior. At its heart, ableism is rooted in the assumption that differently abled people require "fixing" and defines people by their disability. Ableism classifies entire groups of people as "less than," and includes harmful stereotypes, misconceptions, and generalizations of people with disabilities. Stigma ableism manifests for autistic adults in others making assumptions that they are not intelligent or cognitively at their level, not capable of doing a certain type of work or not able to

Table 3.1 Typical ASD Presentations at Home and Work (Rodden, 2020)

HOME PRESENTATIONS	WORK PRESENTATIONS
• Family members lovingly refer to the person as the "eccentric professor" of the family, even though they don't work in academia.	• Having a conversation with a boss and prefer to look at the wall, their shoes, or anywhere but directly into their eyes.
• Always wanted a best friend, but never found one.	• Co-workers say the person speaks like a robot.
• Often invent their own words and expressions to describe things.	• Each item on their desk has a special place and it is not appreciated when it is disturbed.
• Even when they are in a quiet place, like the library, they may make involuntary noises like clearing their throat over and over.	• Really good at math, or software coding, but struggle to succeed in other areas.
• Follow the same schedule every day of the week, and don't like unexpected events.	• Talks to co-workers the same way they talk with family and friends.
• Expressions like, "Curiosity killed the cat" or "Don't count your chickens before they hatch" are confusing to them.	• During meetings, they may make involuntary noises, like clearing their throat over and over.
• Prefer to play individual games and sports, like golf, where everyone works for themselves instead of working toward a common goal on a team.	• When talking with a boss, they have difficulty telling if the boss is happy with their performance or mad at them.
	• May exhibit extraordinary talents in visual skills, music, math, and art.

complete a task, cannot understand, need help with everything, cannot learn, are not at their level, and should be somewhere else (not with the neurotypical population).

Spencer Beard, *The Fine, Underappreciated Art of Breathing*

Spencer Beard is an autistic adult. He is a college graduate and spends time pursuing his career passions of education and writing. When he is not working, he spends time with his friends and family. In his writing (*The Fine, Underappreciated Art of Breathing*) he shares his perspective and experiences about being an adult with autism.

When I was younger, with no one to tell me any the wiser, I hated myself for being autistic. I knew I was different. Don't think that an autistic person can't tell they're different. If anyone tells you otherwise, they either don't know what they're talking about, or trying to sell an evil ideology.

Let me ask you a question. Have you ever played that game where you, and maybe with a couple of friends, held your breath underwater to see how long you could stay down? What was your record? A minute? Two minutes? Maybe three? Could it be that you somehow made it to four?

Guess what, I got you beat. I stayed under for twenty-two years.

Okay, I admit. I did not mean that literally. That was just a heavy-handed metaphor. But hey, I still think I can do that since, either way, I almost died from that. If I didn't make that decision to talk to my parents about counselling after a major existential crisis, I wouldn't be here right now. You might still be reading this book, but not this passage.

Looking back, it was my decision to stay under. Sure, nobody told me that I should've come up, some even suggested that I stay under longer, but if I blamed everyone that didn't tell me to come up, I would be blaming everyone. I don't think that's fair.

In some ways, I should have just accepted how my mind and body reacts to things differently. Let me give you an example of what I mean by that. If you're a neurotypical and you see an opinion on the internet about something you disagree with, I'm going to assume you just replied and moved on. That's the calm way of dealing with different opinions after all.

I, on the other hand, have an absolute fit about it. I shake around, flap my hands, get upset. But with that, comes with extreme self-reflection. Through my fits, I think about why I'm doing this. Am I overreacting? Am I wrong for having my opinion? Do they have an uninformed opinion? Do I? Despite how I look physically while having these fits, they give me a unique thought process that most people don't have.

But I'm not the only one who "does odd behaviors," like flapping my hands when stressed, getting underneath blankets to avoid lights/sensory details, or chewing on chew toys because it feels good. I'm always learning more from other autistics on the internet, and it's comforting knowing that I'm not the only one that does stuff like this.

Even our literalness and our inability to get metaphors, something well-known and mocked, is something that I share pride with other autistics. It's our behavior; it's how our mind works. Besides, my literalness only happens in conversations. When I'm thinking creatively, I do understand them to a point. I even started this essay with one. Honestly, if any of that stuff about me came out in 2016, I would have stopped holding my breath and floated all the way down to the bottom. Now, I'm pretty excited to come up and show off my autism. Now, I didn't even want anonymity for writing this passage. Have my autistic name. I live autistically, as there is no other way for me to live.

With everything I have said, you might be surprised that, at the time of this writing, I not only have a job, I have three. I have two jobs that are online, both from the same company. This company, which focuses on teaching composition to homeschool students, requires me to grade students' work, explain what the student did well and didn't do well, and communicate with the students through email over any issues. My third job, where I work as a librarian assistant, I assist the librarian with whatever she needs, or with whatever my patrons need. If the librarian is gone, I become the de facto librarian. Everything in the library would have to go through me.

Were you surprised to hear about my responsibilities? I know I have sensory issues, but I can lead life happily on my own terms. People rely on me every day, and people learn valuable life skills from me every day. In fact, I believe my sensory issues are part of what let me get this far in life. I wouldn't even describe them as "issues," that's just too insulting to myself and what I do.

To help balance that with my differences, I consider myself part of a "mental minority." I am disabled, but my disability is invisible. I can work, but society is not designed for autistics. But I can live with that. I wouldn't trade my autism for the world.

As I am writing this, it's late, I should've been in bed an hour ago. I gotta get up at 6:45 A.M. for my job, ready for a full day's work. I'm still minorly reeling from a break-up I initiated months ago, looking for new partners to be with, planning various projects, thinking about how to schedule my online jobs more wisely, and writing some very personal creative works.

I get up. I take a deep breath of air, while standing on the beach of hope with the ocean of doubt waving back and forth behind me. I look at the horizon of the rising sun.

Today is gonna be a great day.

Common Struggle Areas

Independent living ability often highlights the struggles that autistic adults encounter. Independent living encompasses many things and can look differently for each person with autism. In general, independent living ability refers to the ability of an individual to function in adult life on their own without an accommodation, another person assisting them, doing for them, or making up for some skill need. Some adults may struggle with issues such as being able to manage a budget, grocery shop, cook for themself, manage appointments, or acquire a driver's license. Others may be mostly independent but require an occasional accountability person to make sure they are managing well. Other adults may be severely lacking in independent skills and require full-time care. Severely impaired individuals will likely have co-occurring issues other than autism and likely have been dealing with this level of impairment since childhood. These individuals will also likely be under the legal guardianship of a parent or caretaker.

Adults with ASD, may struggle with building relationships, social navigation, and participating in recreational activities. This can be even more difficult because of a childhood full of social interaction rejection, and the lack of knowledge that most people in the leisure and community services have when it comes to ASD (Sicile-Kira, 2004). Arguably a unifying issue in autism is social functioning. Although the exact social needs will vary from person to person, on some level there is typically a social skill struggle. Depending on the social skills struggles, the autistic adult can have a challenging time navigating adult life and even find themselves in debilitating situations.

Becoming a legal adult at age 18 typically coincides with graduating high school and is considered a time of transitioning to adulthood. Moving into a work life or continuing education at a college or university can be a common next step. For those with ASD both environments hold the potential for struggles. Many colleges and universities do not offer services or offer very minimal services to assist the needs of autistic individuals. As a result, the higher education experience can be a time of great social challenge, communication struggles, and relationship issues. Anxiety levels can be heightened and can negatively affect academic performance.

Work life can often feel intimidating for those with autism. Hendricks (2010) reported that employment statistics for autistic individuals are appalling. Adults experience underemployment, switch jobs frequently, have difficulty adjusting to new job settings, make less money than their counterparts, and are much less likely to be employed than typically developing peers. Autistic Adults encounter many struggles in work life including interactional difficulties, communication and social difficulties with supervisors and coworkers, difficulty understanding directions, inability to "read between the lines," difficulty reading facial expressions and tone of voice, asking too many questions, and communicating in an inappropriate manner. Further, they may experience social impairments which involve a wide array of deficits and can include inappropriate hygiene and grooming skills, difficulty following social rules, inability to understand affect, working alone, and acting inappropriately with individuals of the opposite sex. Those with ASD can also possess high levels of stress and anxiety in the workplace which may interfere with performance.

Sensory processing issues are a typical struggle area for autistic individuals and sensory struggles permeate throughout any environment including work, school, and home. Sensory processing difficulties are defined as a person's system not being able to take in sensory input such as sound, touch, or sight – there is a "traffic jam" in processing and the person becomes highly uncomfortable and dysregulated. Our bodies are consistently receiving sensory messages and thus, difficulties with sensory processing can affect every part of an adult's life. Sensory processing challenges are one of the primary symptoms in receiving an autism diagnosis and many adults with ASD struggle with sensory challenges.

Research has identified that around 80–85% of adults with autism indicate they have some challenges with sensory processing. Research has also identified that sensory processing challenges contribute to an adult's increased levels of stress. For those with autism, the larger and more unpredictable the environment, the more sensory input there is for the autistic adult to process and possibly experience challenge.

Many struggles autistic individuals encounter are with and/or about other people's intolerance and socially rigid expectations. Shore (2003) highlighted in an excerpt from *Beyond the Wall: Personal Experiences with Autism and Asperger's syndrome,* some of the challenges in navigating life as an autistic adult:

After receiving my bachelor's in Music Education and Accounting & Information Systems I set forth to work in a medium sized Certified Public Accountants firm. Boy was that a mistake. I went to work at an accounting firm, from which I was let go after three months.

I spent hour after hour preparing financial statements by hand for the auditing of mutual funds; so much so that I got tendonitis of the wrist. As the low man on the totem pole, I would spend much time verifying the work others had done. Even though I had just graduated as an honors student with a bachelor's degree in the field, I often felt my coworkers were talking in another language when they explained procedures and where different documents were located. It seemed as if I had been dropped into a foreign culture. I felt like I needed to be shown step by step in a discrete manner to get a grasp of what was expected of me. No one was willing to do that for me.

I was closely supervised and was expected to fit in with all of the accountant/business employees. The business uniform is the suit and tie... which drove me nuts. I can't stand to wear a tie. The only way I could survive was to ride my bicycle from where I lived (about 7 miles) to work and enjoy the out-of-doors for an hour and a half each day. It took 45 minutes to get to work this way as opposed to the 2 hours by public transportation. Made sense to me.

Riding my bicycle to work and changing into my suit in the basement of the office was too weird for them. The personnel officer told me that I had better take public transportation and arrive at the office in my suit. Thinking back to that time I realize that I could not have chosen a place that was more conservative, and conformist had I tried. Probably all financial institutions are like this. After a while I spent most of my time in their library reading business reference books as the supply of work seemed to dry up. On occasion, I would seek out work from other coworkers, or drop into one of the senior manager's office for a chat.

An assignment with a fellow accountant at the firm didn't work out well at all. I could never really understand what he wanted, and he seemed irritated at the things I did. The bank where we worked was overheated. In response to that I would often open the window and take off my shoes when I was sitting at the desk out of view of other people. He didn't like that at all. While auditing a ledger I mentioned to him that it was difficult to read some of the numbers.

One day the personnel officer called me into his office and told me he was letting me go. He said that I just didn't seem to fit in and suggested that there may have been a disability that I had failed to disclose to him when I interviewed for the job. That disability may very well have been there. To me, however, it was something of the past and it never occurred to me that accommodation may have been needed. I just thought I was stupid because I didn't "get it." Getting fired was very humiliating and embarrassing to me. With a fuzzy, heavy feeling in my head I gathered my belongings and left.

My next job was at a large bank as a portfolio accountant. I made trades for, received interest and dividends for, and created regular financial reports for $750,000,000 of pension fund money. I had now learned better how to blend into the business world. They tolerated my riding my bicycle to work. However, I was miserable being involved in the business culture.

In addition, the assumption that I had left the bullies behind in junior high school, was incorrect. They were here too. Save for friends from India and Ethiopia, I kept to myself. I simply was not interested in spending the day yacking about team sports and how much a certain couch cost. I stayed at this large bank for the next year and a quarter but was unhappy there. I love the study of business, accounting and taxation but I cannot stand working with the people who choose these areas for their careers.

I left this job after 15 months to teach business at the vocational and college level. The strange thing is, that I find the STUDY of business, taxes, the stock market, etc. fascinating. I also enjoy TEACHING business subjects, but not as much as teaching music. I just can't tolerate working with the personality types who are attracted to this field.

A Better Fit

I realized that teaching was for me. There was no close supervision with someone watching my every move. My supervisors and students were closer to accepting me as myself then in any previous position. They actually respected that I rode my bicycle to work. My next place of employment was at a finishing school for secretaries. A warning like what is issued by the robot on the TV show Lost in Space should have gone off in my head: Too strict a dress code... I was let go from that place after two years.

The Best Fit

When I got my job as professor of music and computers in January 1994, I knew I had found my niche. I could do what I loved and expend much less energy trying to blend in. As long as students are happy, learning what they are supposed to, the administration is happy too.

There are some people there who respect what I do for the school and serve as mentors. They inform me of potential political blunders I may be about to make and are ready to help bail me out if I get into trouble. It is often difficult for me to read the political wind of things and I'm terribly susceptible to bully-types that cross my path.

Those of us in the Fine and Performing Arts are frequently expected to be somewhat quirky and that suits me fine! By the way, I don't have to wear a tie! Some people at work may sense that I'm different but most of the school community has no true sense of what I'm really about.

After this trip through various places of employment some things became clear to me. To survive as a full-time employee of an organization, these tenets must be followed by me.

1. I must know myself well enough to know where in the workplace I fit in. I seriously misjudged that as I entered the business world. The conformity along with the suit & tie thing just doesn't work for me.
2. Close supervision of my day-to-day activities doesn't work for me. I do much better if I'm given a task and a period of time to figure out what must be done, usually in a way that it hasn't been done before.
3. Find a mentor or mentors I can trust. They can save your employment life.
4. Having an interest in a particular field doesn't mean that it is good for me to work in.
5. There is more to life than work. [Really?] Yup! I'm still learning that.

Supporting Adults with ASD

Gerhardt (2004), communicated that any system of intervention or support for an autistic individual needs to identify the individual, environmental, instructional and community conditions where an individual with ASD can experience success without stigmatization. Using this perspective, the autistic adult becomes simply one target of potential intervention among a variety of targets (coworkers, modifications to job requirements, the physical environment, etc.) designed to support increasingly greater levels of personal independence and competence. In this model, the goal is not to "fix" the adult with ASD but rather to simply view them as one of many potential targets for instruction, support and growth, and in doing so, reduce the impact of potentially debilitating barriers which increases personal competence of all involved.

One of the simplest ways to support an autistic adult is to ask them how they can be supported. Talking to the person, getting to know them, building a relationship with them, and inquiring about what would make their life easier and what supports might help them is fundamental to being supportive and autism friendly. Some additional points for being supportive include:

- be willing to ask autistic adults questions when you do not understand something. Take notes on things you do not understand and be willing to listen and learn,
- ask about and learn all you can about how the person's ASD affects them being sure to respect privacy and what the person wants to talk about and share,
- understand communication systems may be different for each of you and assist the person with ASD in developing a workable communication system,
- do not focus on weaknesses but discover and appreciate the strengths of the person with autism,
- provide polite persistence and respectful reminders when addressing issues with the autistic person,
- be an ally, someone the person with ASD can feel comfortable approaching and asking about social situations and how to navigate scenarios,
- help the autistic person create a "life folder" that contains visual representation for important things to remember. This can be names, phone numbers, and processes and protocols. It can be work-specific or life in general,
- support the autistic adult in developing self-advocacy skills,
- for work and higher education settings, establish a special department to assist with the needs of those with autism,
- explore some basic advocacy work,
- and learn about the person's rights under the Americans with Disabilities Act (ADA) and help them acquire accommodations.

Recognizing Strengths in Adults with ASD

An autistic adult can possess many strengths that can be utilized and valued in adult life. Many individuals with autism can be desirable employees because of strengths that are common in those with ASD such as attention to detail, perseverance on repetitive and monotonous tasks, ability to adhere to highly structured tasks that involve a lot of rules, and enthusiasm for tasks in their area of special interest (Rosenblatt & Carbone, 2019).

Grandin (2012) highlighted that autistic individuals often have special interests or obsessions in which they are often well versed, knowledgeable about, and able to execute effectively. These special interests can be developed into an employable skill. Even though social interaction skills may be lacking, talent, strength, and ability in a special interest area can be valued and admired for work success. Having a special ability can convince others that the individual is worthy of employment. Autism friendly professionals can recognize and advocate for awareness of the positive attributes that those with ASD possess.

Russell et al. (2019) reported that autistic individuals do possess several strengths including the ability to hyperfocus, attention to detail, good memory, and creativity skills. Additional skills noted included specific qualities relating to social interaction, such as honesty, loyalty, and empathy for animals or for other autistic people. A myriad of research has supported that people with ASD have remarkable strengths in the areas of memory, accuracy, concentration, and problem solving. In some cases, people with autism have extraordinary strengths and talents in music, visual art, and calendar counting (Miller, 1999).

Strengths become more important depending on the environment the adult is in and how necessary it is to possess a strength. Many employers may hire autistic adults due to their attention to detail – they can look at code and quickly find errors, they are able to design and build structures that are safe and typically require fewer revisions and may make fewer mistakes than their neurotypical peers. Colleges and universities may be interested in recruiting more students with ASD due to their amazing memory skills, stability and consistency, and the diversity of thought they bring into the classroom. Tech companies may be drawn to the strong visual learning style of autistic individuals as well as their strong connection and comfort with technology. Additional strengths that would be valued in certain settings include concrete thinking, non-emotional responses, and rule and regulation adherence. Understanding that strengths exist and recognizing strengths that commonly amalgamate with an autism diagnosis is a primary example of being an autism friendly professional.

Adulthood provides a perfect canvas for those with ASD to highlight and be valued for their strengths. Adulthood for autistic individuals needs to be understood as more than just a chronological state. For all persons, adulthood represents a time in one's life where there are increased levels of independence, choice, and personal control. Further, adulthood is generally recognized as a period of increased responsibility, commitment, and, often, delayed gratification. It is during this time of life that we generally experience our greatest successes as well as some of our greatest difficulties. Adulthood, despite some popular perceptions, is a time of continued growth and learning and not a period of stagnation, and is, in many ways, the defining period of one's life. Childhood may be looked back on fondly, but it is accomplishments as adults which are generally the most reward-ing. Adulthood for the adult with ASD should be viewed as no different (Gerhardt, 2004).

Ray's Story

Background – Ray was diagnosed with autism as a preschool child. His parents were divorced, and he lived primarily with his father and visited his mother regularly. Both parents were active with Ray and secured mul-tiple therapies for him throughout his childhood. At the time, Ray was diagnosed with autistic disorder, which would be a level three in impair-ment. Ray attended public school and had an IEP. He received many accommodations and special services at school and in the community. As an adolescent, Ray worked with a nonprofit service dedicated to helping those with ASD acquire job skills and employment. This process did not go well, and Ray was unable to maintain a job.

At age 18, Ray's father took legal guardianship of Ray. As an adult, he continued to live with his father and regularly visit his mother. He was placed on a waitlist for a work program specifically designed for those with greater impairments and after about a year was able to start working in this program. Outside of participating in the work program, Ray's out of home activities consisted of occasionally going somewhere with one of his parents. Ray spent a great deal of time at home online and playing video games. Ray's parents were supportive of him but somewhat at a loss for what Ray could do and be involved with.

Struggle areas – The primary struggle for Ray was his impairment level. This limited what Ray was able to do on his own. He had challenges cognitively and could do only a few things without supervision. Ray's social functioning, processing, and reasoning ability were all impaired. Tasks that were complex, involving multiple steps or problem solving were extremely challenging for Ray. Many of Ray's struggle areas involved interacting with other people or systems. He was easily confused and often this created dysregulation for Ray.

Strengths – Ray had a pleasant cooperative personality unless he was dysregulated. He had a strong desire to advance and reach goals and was usually willing to participate in new programs or therapies to improve himself. He had a solid vocabulary and could speak well. Ray was knowledgeable and good with video games and navigating technology. This area seemed to come naturally to him and was also enjoyable for him. Ray could independently complete simple one or two step tasks such as walking down the street to a restaurant and buying a meal.

Supports and services – Throughout Ray's childhood he received and participated in multiple services and therapies. Ray had special accom-modations at school and participated in community therapies and support groups. He received a variety of interventions such as behavioral therapy, speech therapy, occupational therapy, social skill groups, and AutPlay® Therapy. As an adolescent, he participated in a job skill development program and independent living classes. When Ray became an adult, many of the services he received as a child discontinued and were not available for adults. Services and supports were minimal for him as an adult. He was able to secure therapy services and eventually be accepted into a work program for those with a greater impairment. Ray was also placed on disability and he was able to receive some services through disability support.

Autism friendly experiences – Ray received support and validation from his parents and some of the therapies he was involved with but overall, he was usually devalued by others (individuals and systems). Ray had clear impairments, and this usually meant others would quickly assess that he was incapable. As an adult, he was often treated like a child. Outside of his immediate family, Ray's autism friendly experience was not good. He encountered a great deal of ableism. Many of these incidents were likely due to a lack of knowledge and misplaced good intentions but they were still hurtful for Ray and he spent time in therapies addressing these issues and working on improving his self-worth.

Ben's Story

Background – Ben was diagnosed with autism as an adolescent. His diagnosis at the time was Asperger's syndrome. He lived with his father and mother and had one younger sister who was neurotypical. Ben had attended public school his whole life and had done well academically. He had some struggles socially in elementary school but nothing that seemed to warrant concern. In junior high and high school, he began having many social challenges and high levels of anxiety which led to an evaluation and diagnosis of autism. Ben did not receive any special accommodations at school and had not participated in any therapies until his diagnosis. His first time entering therapy to address any autism issues was when he was 16 years old.

Ben's parents were supportive of Ben and wanted him to receive help for the issues he was struggling with but were mostly unaware of autism and how it affected individuals. Ben was resistant to the autism diagnosis and felt that it carried an extremely negative stigma. Ben worked on improving his social functioning and graduated from high school and went to college. He struggled socially in college but did well academically and graduated with a degree in engineering. Ben secured a full-time job and had his own apartment and was fully independent. Ben continued to struggle in social situations/relationships and with poor self-worth, primarily associated with his autism. Ben attempted a few relationships, but they ended badly. He struggled in adolescence and adulthood in forming meaningful relationships and feeling ashamed for having autism.

Struggle areas – Ben was a good example of someone with autism who could "pass" as neurotypical. It would be challenging for the casual observer to know that Ben had autism. His primary struggles were related to social functioning. In limited social situations Ben could perform well but in more complicated scenarios such as forming and maintaining a friendship or getting into a romantic relationship, Ben struggled a great deal. These areas in his life were left unfulfilled and Ben experienced a great deal of rejection socially and had built up shame and anxiety about social interactions. The combination of Ben's social anxiety, poor self-worth (related to social functioning), and his autism shame presented the largest challenges for Ben.

Strengths – Ben possessed a plethora of strengths, many that were equal and/or above his neurotypical peers. Ben had a strong vocabulary and academic ability. He was physically athletic and able to navigate many components of his life successfully. Ben possessed a pleasant personality with a good sense of humor. He desired to be successful and possessed a strong work ethic. He was able to live independently without assistance and his family was encouraging and supportive.

Supports and services – Ben did not receive any supports or services for his struggles until he was 16 years old. He began therapy to work on improving his social functioning and decrease his social anxiety. As an adult, Ben continued his therapy and worked to address his poor self-worth issues and his conceptualization of autism as shame. Many services and additional supports that might have benefited him were not explored as Ben did not want to participate in anything that would highlight he had autism.

Autism friendly experiences – Ben did not share with others that he had autism and thus many people that Ben encountered in his life were unaware of this diagnosis. Ben was often rejected socially and had many negative experiences in this area. It is likely most people mislabeled Ben's behavior and interactions and never considered there was an autism issue. Ben's main challenge with autism friendly experiences was the way he treated and viewed himself as a person with autism. Through therapy Ben was able to become more self-actualized about having ASD and dissipate the stigma and shame that he had held onto for many years. The larger autism friendly message is how Ben assessed the culture around him and determined that autism would be viewed as something negative and thus something to keep hidden. The autism friendly professional should consider what messages they are sending that might make those who are differently abled feel shameful and how to reframe with a message that is validating and supportive.

Autistic adults face a myriad of issues. Services and supports dissipate considerably once someone becomes an adult. Independent living and relational deficits become more noticeable and the ability or lack of, to navigate life takes a more serious tone. The adult world is often less forgiving of struggles and mistakes – where a child might be given more grace and latitude, an adult is often judged more quickly and harshly. The autism friendly professional has the opportunity to represent something different from what the adult with ASD is often receiving. An autism friendly professional is always an active ally in creating a supportive space of navigation for autistic individuals.

4 How Autism Affects Families

Just as autism is a spectrum of presentation, families living with autism are also represented across a wide spectrum. Although these families are unified by autism, how the autism affects the family can vary considerably. Monteiro (2016) highlighted that every family navigating their autism journey has their own story to tell, their own family narrative. ASD does not discriminate, families are seemingly chosen at random to welcome a child into their lives who will later be diagnosed with autism. Whether giving birth to a child, adopting, fostering, grandparenting, or taking guardianship, the chances of loving and caring for an autistic child are consistently increasing. This chapter captures an authentic picture of the joys and the struggles of life with autism, highlighting the human spirit and the strength of a family.

The more we learn about families and ASD, the more we understand they have the same stressors as all families, and the autism "stuff" is in addition. Families still get flat tires, pay for braces to straighten their children's teeth, make dinner, celebrate birthdays, and even have jobs. The first thing to understand about a family affected by autism is that they can have the same celebrations and struggles that any family might be experiencing. When focusing on specific struggles with ASD and families, it is essential to understand the everyday mundane challenges that families experience. Often the simple activities of the day that a neurotypical family might navigate can be a stressful, challenging, and an energy draining event for the family with ASD. Grant, Stone, & Mellenthin (2020) reported that parents are often dealing with high levels of stress and frustration with their child and/ or child's condition. Bonis (2016) described the frequency and high levels of stress that parents of children with ASD experience, scoring higher on levels of stress than other groups of parents. Being aware and providing support to someone through words of encouragement and understanding is a welcome gesture, but if a family is struggling to put food on the table or does not have money for gas, then words have little meaning. Families affected by ASD often have basic needs that must be met. These needs are often additionally impacted or compromised because of employment difficulties, financial concerns, and lack of childcare.

DOI: 10.4324/9781003105633-5

Before delving into finances and other stresses we must look at the initial impact of receiving an ASD diagnosis. When a child joins a family as a newborn there is usually limited concern of their development. When a new child is welcomed into a family there is a bonding time and expectations begin to develop. These expectations come in the form of dreams families have for their child. The family may look forward to trips to Disneyland, soccer games, dance classes, and driving lessons. The parents may anticipate weddings and grandchildren in the future. But for children with autism, shortly into the child's life, parents and professionals notice that developmental milestones are not being reached. Often a lack of shared attention, delayed language, and slow overall progress are noticed. At this point families often proceed in a response and reaction – some pursue early intervention programs to try and address the developmental concerns, others proceed with caution, waiting to see if things naturally improve, and some deny there is anything different about their child and ignore the developmental signs. Whether a full diagnosis is made and accepted, or there is simply the realization that their child has struggles beyond those of their peers, for many parents a phase of mourning or grief begins.

The Grief Cycle

Parents of a child diagnosed with ASD are often unexpectedly introduced to a type of grief cycle. There are different versions of grieving, but the Kübler-Ross grief cycle (denial, anger, depression, bargaining, and acceptance) often resonates with families (Gregory, 2020). Each parent, sibling, and other family members will enter and progress through the phases in their own time. The grief cycle is an individualized process and a diagnosis of ASD does not trigger a particular stage for everyone. A person may have worked through the entire cycle quickly and be at the level of acceptance by the time a diagnosis is obtained. A parent could be relieved and ready for a diagnosis and happily affirming of their child with autism. Most family members will not travel through the grief cycle stages together; many times this can cause communication disruptions for family members and extra caution should be taken to recognize this possibility. Each person in the family must travel their own journey and hopefully provide support to one another along the way.

The grief cycle resonates with many parents, as typically an autism diagnosis is a surprise and not what the family expected. Parents must often reframe what they thought their life, their child's life, and their expectations were going to be. When the signs of autism begin to emerge, the first phase (denial) begins. Denial comes in the form of avoidance of the topic, confusion of what is really supposed to be "normal," or a manifestation of fear. It is a form of rejecting the information or situation – it is not real. Denial aids in the pacing of a person's feelings of grief.

Instead of becoming completely overwhelmed with grief, the person denies it, does not accept it, and staggers the full impact. When a diagnosis of ASD is given, shock may become part of the denial scenario. As parents begin to seek answers, there may be a form of elation denial that happens as new pieces of information are discovered that can be perceived as hope and somehow validating the diagnosis is not accurate.

The next phase is anger. Anger may present itself as frustration, disbelief, or a feeling of lack of ability to change things. It may manifest as irritation over the situation, anxiety of how this happened, and questioning of what it means for the life of the child and family. Some families are not able to pass through this stage without damage to relationships and/or they get "stuck" in anger and are unable to process forward through the grief cycle. Blame and guilt often begin to appear during this time. Parents desperately search for answers and for a cause. Parents question how this could happen to their child. Since there is no known etiology, speculation begins on what caused the autism.

Blame can quickly be assigned, perhaps to a partner, their choices, or even oneself. Is it genetic? If so, can one person be blamed? Comments like, "They never did figure out what was wrong with your uncle" or "There is a lot of depression and a couple of learning disabilities on your side of the family" are desperate examples of frustration and the need to understand a reason. The blame might turn inward and result in an intense sense of guilt, feeling anxious that somehow the fault lies within. And, if it is not genetic, who did something wrong? Who made a choice that caused this? What if I had made different choices? These questions pit family members against one another or against a system. A person may be angry at autism. Why did it ensnarl their child? The answer to the question of how can be a consuming, futile, lifelong quest which takes away from the important work of affirming and parenting the autistic child.

Moving to the next phase, a family faces depression. This is the phase when it is realized that an initial dream may be lost. Families may feel overwhelmed, helpless to change or fix what is happening, and even hostile toward professionals, society, and ASD. Some people can move through this phase quickly while others may always cling onto the perceived loss and allow the depression to frame their whole world. A father broken from multiple ASD diagnoses for his two sons sat at his daughter's soccer game, the first one he attended, and wept that he would never see his sons with autism play sports. As a soccer player himself he felt robbed of that shared life experience, robbed of his sons being able to have this experience. As he sat consumed, he missed the smiles of his daughter who was playing to impress him. Although his daughter played soccer for over four years, he never volunteered to help the team, he never went to practice, and he never attended another game. One of his autistic sons grew up and successfully participated in golf and wrestling, yet the father was unable to mutually participate in his children's success. Depression is powerful. It was not the diagnosis of autism that robbed this father of precious family experiences – it was the depression he was unable to conquer.

Once a family begins to grasp that "this autism thing" is not going away, they enter the bargaining phase. They begin to reach out to others through support groups and look for meaning. They begin to share their story as a bridge to others and a cathartic release of built-up emotions. They also begin to reach out to professionals for help and guidance. For others, it is important to be present for this stage of grief without judgement. This is a "figuring it out" stage for families affected by autism. Families are given a plethora of information, some of it conflicting in nature, so they must navigate their experiences to find what is the best fit for their family. Others should remember they have not been in the family's situation and cannot fully understand what it feels like for the family. Nor can an observer know the effort that may have been put into learning a new task, avoiding a meltdown, or decision made to manage day to day life. Often parents will reach out to other parents wanting confirmation that while it is hard, they are doing the best they can, and they are "good" parents. Families may participate in fundraising walks and join support groups to find acceptance and companionship. They will begin to share their stories – the defeats, the sorrows, the joys, and the successes. Autism friendly individuals will listen to what families have to say. They will not try to control the family or compare them to some other family who has it worse or has handled it better. This can be a confusing time for families affected by ASD and they will need genuine autism friendly support to navigate the bargaining phase.

The final stage in the grief process is acceptance. This involves making a new plan and exploring options for a bright future. Acceptance can look like mindful behaviors, engaging with reality as it is, being present in the moment, adapting, coping, and responding skillfully. It can feel like validation, pride, courageousness, and wisdom. One of the best-known descriptions of accepting a disability diagnosis comes from the article *Welcome to Holland* by Emily Perl Kingsley (1987). Kingsley presented the analogy of preparing for a trip to Italy but ending up in Holland. It is a new experience and not the one that was imagined or planned for, but a new trip that can be amazing. When families move into acceptance, they are able to move past a diagnosis, move past limits, and embrace joy and fulfillment in living their life in their reality affirming, cherishing, and supporting their autistic child.

Jennifer Proctor, *A Family's Journey with Autism*

Jennifer Proctor, a busy mother of three (two daughters diagnosed with autism) lives in Southwest, Missouri and shares her family's journey and life with autism including some of their struggles and victories:

When I hear the word "autism," I have so many mixed emotions and thoughts. This especially hits close to home when I am talking to someone who has also been in my shoes. Having twin girls, aged 11 and both with high-functioning autism, brings back the blur of trying to recall the accomplishments and struggles that they have faced along the way. My first thought is that autism is "hard" followed by remembering that autism is also a "blessing." The littlest things we take for granted everyday are so hard for many of these individuals diagnosed with autism. They may struggle with things like holding a pencil correctly, understanding where their bodies belong in space so that they can keep from bumping into things or people, having increased anxiety in crowded or loud places, difficulty with patience, and just making it through the day.

As a parent, I try to put myself in their shoes and remind myself that these things are hard for them so that I can be more understanding and patient with them. Additionally, reminding myself that as the weekly appointments become exhausting for me with just driving back and forth, imagine what it's like for them to continually have to work on skills that are more difficult for them on a daily basis.

With the struggles, regression, setbacks, and lack of patience – I also get to see the wonderful side of autism as well. With the girls now being older, I have seen goals accomplished, milestones met, and more patience for all of us which helps us lead more meaningful lives to the fullest. Early intervention is the key! Attending therapy appointments, doctor appointments, and social events is definitely worth it! Yes, it's exhausting for everyone included but it is what has helped get us to where we are and caused me to see the light at the end of the tunnel. Autism brings out some pretty amazing talents such as drawing, painting, writing wonderful essays, and not being afraid of what the world thinks of you. These are just a few of the success stories that go along with the blessings of autism in my world.

Autism is hard but is also a blessing and I wouldn't change the journey. You learn so much when you enter their world. Seeing through their eyes is quite amazing! Their perspective is simply different and that's okay – it's what makes them so unique!!! As a parent, it truly is a blessing but can be somewhat of a blur on the voyage. I recommend taking pictures and journaling because you will not remember it all, but you will see the light. And when you do, it's worth all the struggles that you have to encounter along the way!

Challenges for Families

Along with the journey of grief, there are many more areas families affected by ASD can struggle to resolve. Blame and guilt can manifest for a variety of reasons and throughout a family's lifetime. Parents sometimes must make split-second decisions that have negative consequences which are not easily undone. A parent may feel pressured (against their better judgment) to let a child do something "just this one time" which turns into a social or behavioral disaster with long-term effects leaving the parent feeling blame and guilt. Blame often manifests for parents from an unequal or divisive understanding of how ASD affects a child and how to approach behaviors. Studying autism and taking children to therapies takes time, and most parents will not have an equal abundance of time to dedicate. This creates an imbalance and a situation where one parent will likely become the expert on parenting the autistic child. It can also develop into a cycle of over-dependence on one parent, or disagreements of how to teach and work with the child. Blame can arise when there is a lack of developmental progression, money is spent on interventions with no results, or behaviors escalate. Parents blame each other for not making the best choice, not listening to the other partner, or for the partner not providing enough help.

Guilt is blame turned inward when a parent feels failure. A large family with multiple children diagnosed with autism had the experience of watching their first diagnosed child learn sign language. This set the family on the path of an incredible journey of accomplishment. The daughter had success signing, even carrying around a sign language book and pointing at objects to learn the signs. The family thought they had found the answer to all things autism. When this child's brother was born, and later diagnosed with ASD, the plan was to duplicate what had been successful for his sister. They would teach him how to use sign language and he would progress as his sister had. Unfortunately, he struggled to get beyond a few basic signs, lacked the fine motor control needed to produce readable signs, and lacked in cooperation skills. The family worked together in full force to replicate what had been done with his sister. In total, he has received more therapies, interventions, and treatments than his two other siblings diagnosed with ASD combined and is still very dependent on assistance for all daily living skills, has very limited speech, and does not read or write. The mother had to work through a great amount of guilt when he did not achieve the same level of skill and independence his siblings enjoy. Once she could process her guilt, she was able to appreciate and enjoy his accomplishments without comparison to the other siblings and without believing she had done something wrong with him. Without the boundary of guilt, the family could celebrate the seeming little things that the world may see as slow progress as great achievements for their son.

Families affected by ASD can provide a multitude of stories and experiences they have encountered from others (many of which are not pleasant or supportive). One young mother, desperate to find a way to get her daughter (pre-autism diagnosis) socializing so she could learn from other children, decided to enroll her in preschool. Following call after call of screening questions, she finally found a place that would at least meet with her. As she was loading her daughter into the car, a pack of candy from the day before was on the seat. Unable to deter her daughter from eating the candy and knowing that taking it from her would send the child into a full-blown meltdown, the mother let her begin to eat the candy. Upon arrival at the preschool, the candy was tightly fisted, and she was not about to let it go. Although the mother would have preferred for the candy to be kept in the car, not wanting to walk in late and not wanting to create a meltdown, a quick decision was made for her daughter to keep the candy. The two were met at the door with introductions and first impression negative assumptions were made about the child and parent. The mother was promptly told a mistake had been made, the appointment would not be happening. Although the mother insisted that a meeting with the director was promised, both mother and child were physically blocked from entering the building and the door was closed as they were left standing just outside the threshold. She left in disbelief holding her only child and feeling completely rejected.

Another mother took her son shopping at a local grocery store. Traveling the aisles with her son, the young child pointed at a shelf and exclaimed in a very loud demanding voice, "I want beans!" In absolute delight, the mother grabbed a can of beans and asked the son if he wanted more. Again, the child repeated in the same voice, "I want beans!" "Yes, dear" was about all his mother could muddle. As the requests continued, an older woman walked by and uttered the words, "I guess teaching manners is not part of this generation." Turning to face the woman and looking her directly in the eyes the mother explained this was a moment to celebrate. This was the first time her son had spoken three words together and she would not let a stranger rob her of this moment of joy. To the woman's credit she changed her attitude, stayed, and celebrated with the mother and son. The woman spent 15 minutes learning sign language and graciously telling the young boy how amazing he was. The mother reflected that this day at the grocery store was the day she learned what it meant to be an advocate for her child.

The preceding stories are two of many that can produce guilt, blame, stress, and highlight struggles that can emerge when raising an autistic child. Although the public world is often a challenge, some struggles are not outside the family but come from within. Relationships between couples can be weakened and even terminated when a family is affected by ASD. It is commonly thought that the divorce rate of couples who have a child diagnosed with autism is much higher than parents of a child without any "special needs." Some research studies have indicated higher divorce rates related to having a child with ASD versus neurotypical children, and other studies have proposed the exact opposite conclusion (Rosenblatt & Carbone, 2019). Rates cannot be compared or even affirmed that autism is the final cause of a divorce. With this variance it is important to not assume partners cannot handle the stress of raising an autistic child. Some couples may progress fine while others may experience relationship struggles. Each family has their own journey and the issues they face will be their own and require the services that are best suited to help them resolve their struggles.

As mentioned at the beginning of the chapter, often couples have an unequal knowledge of ASD. This impacts parenting choices greatly and can cause disruptions in co-parenting and conflicts in decision making. For example, a child might be pushed to act or respond before they have processed a request, and this can cause what seems like defiant behavior, when in fact, it is a slower processing time issue (due to autism). When parents are not on the same page in understanding ASD and how it affects their child, one may jump to swift correction (a practical parenting technique), but the other parent who has studied autism, understands patience is in order. The lack of equal awareness therefore creates a parental imbalance. What about discipline? This is commonly a sensitive subject between parents. A couple may be in agreement before bringing a child into the world, but when they have a child who does not cognitively understand discipline, has sensory issues, or will respond by being aggressive, it changes the planned strategy and now there is disagreement. It is easy to let the stressors and demands of reframing parenting expectations create rifts between a couple.

A key strategy for couples is to have respect for one another's choices and to compromise. For some parents it is easy to get caught up in doing things right and following the plan. It is important for parents to jointly engage in training and understanding of sensory needs, executive functioning, communication techniques, etc. that help with raising autistic children. Grandin (2012) discussed that some of the best training she had as a child which led to the success she is today, was good old-fashioned 60s' manners training and hard work. For couples who are navigating the parenting world of autism – mutual respect, appreciation, and putting in the hard work will take them far in their parenting success and thus, in their relationship.

Another issue for families is navigating the world of autism therapies and interventions. Parents are commonly preyed upon, especially when their children are young, to take part in a cure or a therapeutic or biomedical fix for ASD. Disagreements on what type of interventions to pursue and how to spend limited finances can lead to marital stress. Money is precious during this time because it is attached to how much a child can be helped. Families do not usually have the training to filter through all the potential interventions, tonics, and treatments. A quick internet search will bring up both legitimate and deceptive practices for working with someone on the autism spectrum. Scams, trickery, and illusion are tools that families are faced with as they try to sort the beneficial from the fraudulent. Being on opposite ends of what treatments to pursue can often be a cause of marital discord.

Another point of stress regarding treatment is the constant pressure of providing therapies, interventions, and the associated medical expenses. Some children and adults on the autism spectrum have several additional diagnoses. Parents struggle with intervention decisions and the incurred payments. There are several different approaches parents can access and choices that must be made. There are medical models, holistic approaches, developmental models, behavioral approaches, etc. There can be differences in priorities and desired types of interventions or supports to engage in, causing disagreements among parents. These differences may include acquiring a debt with the possibility of seeing little to no benefit. And even when there is a positive outcome, the financial debt can overshadow the success; leaving the family to struggle in other areas, and no money left for other family needs.

Many years ago, there was an account of a father who had picked a music CD off a store shelf. He looked at it and told himself the purchase of the CD would pay for 15 minutes of therapy, and then he placed it back on the shelf. This simple and powerful analogy highlights the expense of supporting a child with ASD. Therapy (even legitimate, worthwhile therapy) is expensive. Some families do not have insurance and even if they do, insurance does not pay for everything. Special schools and programs can cost a great deal and are usually paid for out of pocket. The expenditure is not only financial, but also time intensive. It is extremely easy for families to be consumed by providing therapy for their child. There are many waiting room visits, waitlists, and time intensive treatment activities. This all prevents families from leading perfectly wonderful boring lives or attending the sibling baseball games, ballet practice, or simply enjoying an agenda-free evening at home.

Obtaining a successful education for their autistic child can become an all-encompassing and stressful experience for a family. School districts and the special education programs they offer can be the determinant for where the family chooses to live. Families often take this information into consideration when choosing a home or deciding to move. While neurotypical families often consider school programs when making decisions, it carries a much greater amount of weight when autism is brought into the equation. Staying with a successful school program versus a job change is a complicated decision. Wanting to move away from a program that is not fulfilling a student's needs is weighed against the needs of other students in the home. Finances complicate the need or desire to possibly relocate or transfer to a private school focused on autism. Many families will change jobs and move for the hope of a better educational experience for their child with ASD. Several families will acquire a second or third job to pay for the tuition to attend an autism focused private school. Educational issues bring about a variety of stressors as families try to navigate learning environments that are not commonly designed for their child.

Sibling Struggles

As children begin to grow and the learning and accepting of ASD is settling on the family, parents begin to focus on the future and siblings. Birth order can influence the path a family makes for themselves. Older and/or neurotypical siblings often find themselves in caregiving roles with expectations of helping younger or differently abled siblings function in the community. A lifestyle change happens when a younger brother or sister with ASD is born. The older neurotypical sibling is no longer a primary focus like most older siblings. But rather than a relinquishing of their attention title, they often exchange it for a heavier workload and increased responsibility. Younger neurotypical siblings quite often have to grow up quickly and take the confusing role of an elder sibling as the skills they are gaining surpass their older sister or brother with autism.

Jealousy is common in families with multiple children. Quite often the foundation of these jealousies is based on an unfair division of attention, time, and resources. When adding an ASD diagnosis to this dynamic, the factors contributing to jealousy are multiplied. Parents are forced to make choices to provide necessary autism-specific support at the cost of a sibling's childhood expectations. It is very tricky to maneuver through this gantlet of needs. One family made the decision to make the "autism things" about needs and respecting each other, not about autism. Children were reprimanded because they made their sibling cry, not because they did not make allowances for their ASD. They also taught siblings to be patient and kind because their brother or sister cannot speak up for themselves, not because they have ASD. As parents they never said we cannot do this or go there because your sibling has autism. It was not always easy for the family and not always successful but overall worked well. Families affected by autism take many paths in managing sibling-related issues, needs, and struggles. It undoubtedly takes time, attention, and resources away from a neurotypical sibling to raise a child with recurring appointments/therapies who also needs help with daily living skills. The feelings siblings have of unfairness or rejection are real. Rosenblatt & Carbone (2019) proposed that siblings can experience tremendous stress and resentment. Many siblings experience a mix of emotions, feeling loving and supportive one minute, angry and bitter the next. Providing siblings an outlet for their emotions and helping fill the voids they are experiencing can make a huge difference in their lives and their feelings toward their autistic sibling.

Neurotypical siblings are charged with some specific duties. They become the eyes and ears at school. They give medication and monitor eating. They protect and they teach. They are also expected to be understanding and place their needs and wants second. They are punched and expected to take it. They bleed and are not allowed to seek revenge. They become parentified. They do all this while mourning the loss of their expected sibling relationship, never realizing in their early years that likely they will one day be asked to be a caregiver or guardian of their sibling with autism. But it can be a beautiful thing to behold a family who works together making their way through life. Some siblings embrace their role as caregiver and best friend. Others become the best cheerleaders shouting out and reporting what new things their sibling accomplished that day. Some relish in the ability to play with and help their sibling with the practice of new skills.

It is important that siblings do not ignore ASD or that there is a family member with autism. ASD should not be a taboo subject, but it does not have to be the main subject. Siblings are given a front row seat to autism and need to have at least a basic understanding of how autism affects their sister or brother. Lack of understanding and knowledge can breed misconceptions, anger, and confusion. Parents must decide how to best approach having autism conversations in the family. The parent must educate, but not in a consuming manner. It is quite easy to let ASD take over the life of a family. It demands attention. But as families grow, they are tasked with creating a delicate balance. Many autism experts suggest that an autism focus should not encapsulate the family's life and instead should be thought of in a percentage such as no greater than 30% or 40% of the family's focus. Families should strive to achieve a healthy ratio that works best for them. There will be times when families are focused on ASD but returning to a balance can keep family life in perspective.

How to be fair to all the children in a family and attend to all their needs, activities, and pursuits is not always easy. As siblings age, often things change. Some identify with being a sibling of a person with autism. They take that charge very seriously and work at creating a strong bond and being an active support person. Others do not want their lives to be defined by being a sibling of a person with a disability; they may be a truly virtuous and caring brother or sister but they want their own lives and not to be a caregiver. Still others may be consumed with worry their own children will have an ASD diagnosis and find that distancing themselves from their sibling is an effective coping mechanism.

However a sibling's feelings manifest, they should be valued and heard and helped to understand they are a sibling of an autistic person. Many siblings discover a place of peace and contentment being a sibling of a sister or brother with ASD. They will likely experience many things as a sibling, such as being embarrassed because an orange their brother carries around ends up in the orchestra pit, taking charge during a seizure while cradling their sibling's head to administer rescue meds, throwing a washcloth over the body parts they do not want to see as they wash their sibling's hair, enjoying getting to hold onto cartoons a little longer than most, and listening to the sounds of someone who is just happy they are around. Siblings can benefit from autism friendly professionals being a supportive person for them and taking the time to listen and learn about their unique lives.

Extended Family Issues

The struggles families endure are not just confined to the boundaries of their home and immediate family relationships. Extended family members play an important role in the emotional, psychological, and social development of autistic children (Grant, 2015). There are often challenges associated with extended family members. Large or small, near or far, extended family members often play into the equation. Some will be supportive from the beginning and may be the first people to suggest that there are developmental concerns. Some will be less supportive, doubting there are any real issues even after a diagnosis. Occasionally extended family issues are based in jealousy. There are thoughts that the ASD family is trying to draw attention to themselves, being dramatic, or excusing behaviors of their child. Some of the most noticeable behaviors of autism can bring on the judgement of those who see or hear them the most. Miscommunication, stares, and off-handed comments by family members can allude to ASD behavior as inappropriate and the result of a spoiled or undisciplined child, thus leaving the parent to feel judged by those who should be their closest support system. As a diagnosis comes, some extended family members will embrace the moment and offer support, while others will doubt the efficacy of the diagnosis and continue to doubt the parenting skills of their family members. There can also be questioning and judgement about the choices made by ASD families concerning therapies and treatments, further driving contention and division within families.

Family members trying to help may offer advice. Although well intended, and possibly well received, it is often unsolicited. These attempts at help are often complicated by the misunderstanding of what ASD really is and not knowing that the spectrum is so varied. In most cases if advice is given to a parent about a child with autism, they have already tried it many times and found that it did not work. Occasionally there can be a helpful piece of advice. A woman, after listening to a friend's concerns about her son's low water consumption, told her she adds ice to all her own child's drinks. As it melts, the water is unwittingly consumed. This was excellent advice for the woman, she tried it and it worked. Often parents of autistic children have had to throw common-sense parenting out the window early on and some of the tricks of the trade are lost. Too often though advice is not asked for or needed, especially from extended family whose love and support should come without condition.

There is typically a lot of pressure on families with an autistic child to conform to behavior expectations during family gatherings. Actions such as leaving the bathroom door open, touching all the food in the potluck buffet, and not taking part in the family activities can make some people uncomfortable, perhaps even causing some to overcompensate. It is easy for autism families to begin to separate themselves from extended family members. It can be the result of not fitting in, exhaustion from being the center of attention, or the sheer effort it takes to be present. Conversations at family gatherings range from soccer games, vacation plans, car preferences, home designs, and reminiscing about great times. Families affected by autism can find themselves very distant from those conversations. Their minds are focused on therapy and how to pay for it, IEP goals, and plan deadlines. This causes them to lose track of what is new and trending and what their neurotypical family members might be pursuing. They have different priorities that are not so easily shut off to join in the basic family conversations. Many families affected by autism remain silent on the struggles they face and instead focus on making sure their child is staying calm and regulated and not disrupting any other family members until they can leave the family event and feel relieved it is over.

Extended family events can vary in their expectations and difficulties. But for many families affected by autism there is always a hypervigilant need for focus and planning. Not all situations are due to uncaring family member responses; some actually involve helpful intentions. For instance, during one holiday meal at Grandma's house, cousins joined in encouraging a highly sensory sensitive child to try mashed potatoes. To the cheers and smiles of cousins she took a fateful bite. She then gagged and vomited across the table. Her mother felt distressed that she had pushed her daughter to meet everyone's expectations. She quickly made her a sandwich and promised her that she would never pressure her again to face such a challenge with an audience. Some family events display the power of how helpful the extended family members can be. A young mother attended her brother's wedding, which was held in a sizable but intimate setting. The young mother's autistic son was overjoyed at the event and far from quiet. Many happy and loud sounds rang from his slender frame. Knowing this moment did not belong to him, but rather to the happy couple, the mother slipped out the door with her son. Seen by the venue security, they were swiftly invited to a room full of security cameras. Viewing the ceremony behind the scenes was not what she had planned for the day but was a happy outcome. Nothing needed to be said or explained to the family. This was a moment of acceptance by all, demonstrating how to do ASD as a family.

Often the child with autism must navigate a different set of rules and practices. This can be noticed by the child and by other family members. Is it fair to the cousins that the autistic child gets to eat his dessert first or watch videos during family time? Why can the family not afford to bring gifts for everyone and bring their fair share of food, or pitch in for the surprise anniversary party? It is a complicated and often taxing mix, resulting in many families attending fewer events and forgetting what it is like to be part of an extended family. While there are many struggles with the dynamics of extended family, it is important to try to capture what can be a future of support and love and how extended family members can aid and provide a source of safety and peace for the family affected by ASD. Cousins can extend the friendship circle throughout an autistic person's life. Uncles and aunts can provide support not only to the child with ASD but also to the parents. Grandparents can be a needed support in helping children get to appointments and providing respite care. Extended family members should look for the opportunity to be on the front lines of being the example of autism friendly.

Daily Home Struggles

As simple as it may seem, sleeping can become a large issue in a family affected by autism. Often, when sleeping and ASD are mentioned, sleep problems are identified as a trigger point of stress for parents. Lack of quality sleep and inconsistent schedules are typical problem areas for a person with autism, but a deeper understanding of how they impact the family should not be overlooked. Parents may find themselves co-sleeping with children for years just so they can get some rest. They may take turns watching their child and monitoring nighttime activities. Their workday can be affected by poor sleep. A person with ASD might be awake during the night (not binge watching their favorite shows) but walking out the front door, eating an entire bag of apples, turning on the stove, and in general being loud. Alone time for parents and retiring to bed together can easily become a distant memory or a point of contention.

There are often complications with sleeping and sleep arrangements. Sleep disturbances and sleep/wake phase complications can plague families. It is one of the primary struggles families complain about. It impacts the whole family's quality of sleep and their productivity during the day. The person who does not sleep is not always demanding attention or disturbing those who are resting, but the quiet night owl is just as worrisome. They could easily be doing something which puts themselves and the family at risk and they are of course hurting their own need for sleep. Families often resort to locks, alarms, co-sleeping or having someone stand watch. Each of these choices changes the natural sleep pattern of the family and can create additional problems.

A family was struggling with their autistic teen son who would not sleep at night. This had been going on for a few years and the family was at a breaking point. The son would seemingly go to sleep at a normal time and the rest of the family would follow. He would easily wake up a few hours later and leave the house and roam around the community, typically looking in trash bins and finding items that he would bring back to his house. The family were often awakened by the police, who would find the teen and bring him back to their home. The family tried many interventions to address this issue, but nothing seemed to work. It became a serious sleep and safety problem for everyone involved and finally the family had to resort to putting several locks and alarms around the house preventing the child from being able to leave the home in the middle of the night. It was not the way they wanted to live but needed to out of desperation. Sleep deprivation leads to a great many things that decrease a person's quality of life. It can impact communication, increase misunderstanding, increase irritability and frustration, create depression-like symptoms, and decrease patience and tolerance levels. Families may need autism friendly support to help troubleshoot sleep deprivation and sleep struggles issues. If this issue is left unaddressed it can easily lead to mental health problems.

ASD can influence and change many things about how the home environment operates. Some of the unforeseen or unknown realities of autism in the home come from property destruction. A child might be continuously picking and peeling things, putting holes in the wall, tearing clothing, ripping papers, and the ever-popular breaking electronics and shattering screens. Most of these actions result in lost items and the expense to replace them. Food preparation becomes a daily issue, fight, or burden, due to sensory or preference restrictions of the family member with ASD. There are often dietary concerns, whether due to specialized diet plans or intolerances. If there are additional family members with dietary needs, especially food allergies, there can be a need for multiple different meals prepared throughout the day. This involves time and expense. A great deal of time is centered around food. When taking in all the considerations and needs of a family with ASD, it is easy to understand how the food preparer can feel like an overwhelmed short-order cook taking away from other family time and experiences.

It can be difficult to clean and maintain a household. There is significantly less time to clean, repair, and replace. There are also struggles with the actual cleaning process; sensory issues that arise from the noise of vacuums, the smell of cleaning solutions, and a child's strong resistance to having things moved from their customary spot. Families must be careful about leaving any toxins accessible, including laundry detergent. Due to sensory issues, the typical safeguards of noxious smells or bitter tastes that deter most people are lacking, causing a person who processes these sensory areas differently to view smelling or drinking these products as not offensive, but rather a delight, putting them in danger. As a person ages, the locks securing these items might not be as effective, so more creativity is necessary to keep loved ones safe and this typically becomes an ongoing, constantly monitored process.

Simple home maintenance that most of us take for granted must be prioritized to keep the person with autism safe. The temperature of the hot water heater might have to be lowered from what is a customary setting, because an autistic person may not regulate their water temperature and scald themselves. Spoiled food must quickly be disposed of out of the refrigerator and moldy bread from the cabinet so as not to be eaten. Lighting may have to be routinely adjusted to address visual sensory issues and certain sounds may have to be avoided, such as starting the dishwasher only when the child is out of the house to avoid noise sensory issues. Specialized doors and windows are sometimes needed to keep flight- risk children safe. While a similar version of some of these issues might be common tasks of neurotypical families, many families with autism must be hypervigilant and often take precautions and organization to an extreme degree to keep things functioning smoothly at home.

Many families have household pets. This can be a positive experience, or it can be a disaster. When a pet is a trained therapy or emotional support animal, it might be a great benefit for the autistic child and even untrained pets can provide companionship and emotional support. Individual personalities of pets and their heightened senses can mesh well with certain family members. One home had a cat that was helpful in alerting to seizures. They also had a puppy that would remain motionless when getting attention from a young voiceless child who could not tolerate typical puppy behavior. The puppy could remain still until the boy was finished petting and would wait for a signal and again become a bouncy baby dog. Although pets can often be helpful, they can also be unpredictable, and it cannot be assumed a person with ASD will welcome a new pet or accept a pet that is already in the home. Introducing a pet into the family and to the child with autism should be a careful, mindful process to ensure a successful experience. Pet shop owners, dog breeders, rescue shelters, etc. can strive to be autism friendly by understanding that the process should be evaluated carefully and work with families on success strategies.

The daily routine and schedule of a family can also be influenced by an ASD diagnosis. Typical routines and decisions throughout the day feel the pressure of autism. One example involves a family's daily morning routine. The son will not leave the house without his morning bath (a ritual the son must perform). Looking ahead to when he is an older man who may still struggle with cleaning himself after toileting, the family decided to keep this ritual, considering that baths and proper hygiene are an important skill. The morning bath ritual creates some issues (the family often sacrifices their timeline) and the family must always plan ahead. Despite the issues, it is a routine with benefits and is identified as a priority for this family. Bath time is assisted and must be supervised due to possible seizures. The son is unable to shower because of sensory issues with water hitting his face. Once dressed and ready to go, the son feels he must make a thorough inspection of the home to be sure everything is in order. Jackets are put on, even though it is 95 degrees outside, then removed again once in the car. Child locks on the door are engaged even though he is 17 years old, as he learned how to get himself out of the car, which he quickly generalized to every time the car stopped including stoplights, stop signs, and waiting for a parking place. This is how each morning must begin for this family, regardless of where they are going or when they must be there. There is little to no room for error or the result could be a behavioral meltdown with farther reaching consequences.

Another example involves a mother's experience with grocery store shopping. The mother, due to not having adequate childcare, would take her son to the grocery store when he was young. He seemed to enjoy going to the grocery store; he especially loved the visual stimulation of the rows of food. But the mother quickly discovered that if something was removed from a shelf and the pattern was disrupted, this would trigger a full meltdown of inconsolable screaming until the item was replaced and the pattern restored. Many months were spent with the mother trying to desensitize and decode this reaction. First, items were taken from the shelf when he was not looking and placed under a blanket. These were short trips with few items that could be slipped to the cashier so he would not notice them being removed from the basket. As time went on the basket load was fuller and the transition to the cashier was accepted. After months of this process the mother was able to remove the blanket, but he still could not tolerate seeing the removal of items from the shelves. Being stifled at this seemingly insurmountable barrier, an idea was generated. He needed to understand the food he had at home came from the grocery store. He loved eating the purchased food when he got home but could not make this connection. One day the mother spoke to the manager of a small grocery store and asked if they would help with the mother's plan and fortunately the store manager agreed to help.

During the next grocery store trip, the mother tried taking some food off the shelves, opening it, and eating it with her son right there in the store. Concluding their shopping, they paid for the items and continued to eat them on the way home, finishing them after they walked into the house. The connection was made. The son understood that people get food from the grocery store and take it home to eat. It took about seven months for the mother to work on this issue and establish a strategy, but the strategy worked, and the mother and son never had another problem at the grocery store. Thankfully, the mother was supported by an autism friendly store manager who agreed to work with her on her plan instead of judging her as an inept parent. Families affected by autism are often reframing the parenting rules. They are the closest thing to being an expert about their child, and this expertise typically comes with a great amount of time and energy, slowly incorporated into daily decisions and practice that may look differently from a neurotypical family but are necessary and successful for the family affected by ASD.

Child Safety Issues

Safety issues can be a reoccurring concern for families affected by autism. Sometimes a child cannot self-report when there is a problem, or when something has happened to them; they may lack the verbal ability or the cognitive understanding. Other times it might be assumed the child does not have the ability to accurately report information and their efforts may be dismissed. This becomes especially difficult when considering health and injury issues. After nine months of looking for reasons why their 12-year-old was not growing, the child was diagnosed with Crohn's disease. The family met with specialists, who could not believe the boy was not reporting pain. Did he not report it, was his way of reporting not validated, or did he not interpret the pain? They will never know, and all could be a possibility.

There are many times when someone self-reports a difficulty or need for assistance and they unwittingly give the listener the opportunity to pass judgement and make assumptions. A woman sat at a dental appointment with her completely independent adult daughter. Because of oral sensory issues, her daughter asked the mother to come along for support. After struggling with the procedure, she confessed to the hygienist that she had sensory issues. This disclosure was met with understanding, which enabled her to feel safe enough to further disclose her ASD diagnosis, which she rarely did. The ASD information was immediately met with the professional turning to the mother to act as the daughter's voice. Disappointed, rejected, and humiliated, the young woman left that office seeing the world as she had feared: It is not always safe to reveal what you are thinking, feeling, and experiencing.

Too often things that are treatable or that need a different approach are missed due to the assumption it is because the person has autism. Exaggerated behaviors are blamed on puberty and ASD, missing many issues that need attention. Parents express concerns of not being taken seriously or the misjudgment that they are grasping for answers or seeking miracles. With multiple diagnoses, parents often find themselves divided between treatment protocols and specialists. One family finds it difficult to treat their son's seizures because he vomits up medication, making it impossible to monitor medication intake and putting him more at risk by administering it. No amount of talking or reasoning will make sense to him as to why he should have to tolerate medication multiple times a day, and his sensory reflex will not allow for him to keep it down. Attempts at explaining this to professionals have been met with disbelief; the parent is not trying hard enough, or the parent is exaggerating.

Safety concerns also manifest when the child ventures outside of the family home and into the care of others. This can be an educational setting, a medical appointment, visiting a friend, participating in church, etc. Often parents fear how their child will be addressed, cared for, and treated by other individuals. There are countless reports of adults who care for autistic children who physically abuse the children, are verbally abusive, and generally mistreat the children. This can also be a concern when children with ASD are around other peers, especially when the scenarios are not supervised by an adult. One of the primary ways autistic children experience a trauma response is from bullying received from peers. Hoover (2015) reported that autistic children are bullied more often than peers with other disabilities and more often than non-disabled peers, those with intellectual disabilities alone, and their typically developing siblings. Children with ASD may lack the ability verbally or cognitively to communicate that someone is mistreating them. Further, even if they have the verbal and/or cognitive ability, they may not understand they are being mistreated and may believe this is the way they are supposed to be treated and thus not tell their parents.

Talking About Autism

Families often struggle with how and when to have discussions about autism. When should a parent tell their child they have an ASD diagnosis? How do they explain autism – what is too much information and what is not enough? Should they consult a professional to help explain ASD to the child? Parents are faced with making the decision of when and how the discussion takes place – or if it will ever happen. Some parents are open about ASD from the beginning and are regularly talking with their child and providing information. Others wait for questions from their child, and yet others hope they will never need to talk about it and want to avoid any labels. Some families care for loved ones who may not be able to cognitively grasp the concept of an ASD diagnosis and thus the conversation is not necessary. Rosenblatt & Carbone (2019) contended that having an open and honest discussion about autism at a level that children can understand is critical to helping the child, siblings and others understand. One key in deciding to discuss ASD is knowing if the information will be beneficial or not to the child. If a child is becoming more and more depressed, even suicidal, because they do not feel they fit in or have friends, it might be more conducive to let them know about their diagnosis, how it affects them, and seek professional help. Many autistic children feel different and notice they are different and interpret this as there is something wrong with them and they are defective. Understanding ASD and providing a concrete reason for their identified differences can be empowering to children with autism.

Many individuals with an ASD diagnosis have additional issues or co-occurring diagnoses. Some are apparent and others are discovered along the journey. Autism can sometimes hide or overshadow other diagnoses. For several years, a family did not see a difference between ASD behaviors and a possible ADHD diagnosis. An incident when they could not get their child to walk down some stairs because he was so distracted began to help them understand there might be issues besides ASD happening. Reaching the latter elementary years and into middle school, they could see the child's disinterest or disengagement turning into a lack of ability to focus long enough to accomplish tasks. This finally led to evaluation and receiving an ADHD diagnosis which was co-occurring with his ASD and thus began specific interventions to help with ADHD struggles. Further, the family had to conceptualize discussing and explaining not only ASD but also ADHD.

This brings up a complication that is fueled by the autism spectrum. The fact that the autism spectrum covers a wide and varied population of people makes it impossible for the observer to have a generalized reaction. This, in part, is where disclosure comes in. Disclosure is when a person's diagnosis is made known. Self-disclosure is when a person discloses this information about themselves. A parent may also choose to disclose information about their child and any diagnosis or issue the child is experiencing. As our communities and the world as a whole move toward inclusion and an acceptance of neurodiversity, it is arguably more important to focus on identifying needs, rather than on deciphering clues to a diagnosis or label. In the dental office the young woman needed the hygienist to slow down and do no more than was necessary. The young woman needed to be able to explain this, and the hygienist needed to hear it without placing a judgment such as treating the woman like a child. None of the functional pragmatics of this important exchange would have been understood by the hygienist simply knowing the woman had autism.

Disclosure is very personal to an individual and/or a family. When does it become about autism? Is it needed or is it obvious? Is a diagnosis something someone proudly shares because they embrace it as part of who they are? Is it not shared for fear of stigmatization? Knowing about ASD makes it possible to support a person and family without the need to know if there is an official diagnosis. We can reach out to others and offer support and kindness without needing a specific diagnosis to do so. People can learn to recognize needs and determine how they can help. An article that was published 25 years ago in a newspaper told the story of a family that was met with scorn in a store checkout line. The family used food stamps to purchase a beautifully decorated cake. A fellow shopper made efforts to humiliate the family by insisting they did not deserve to spend this allotment that way and it was a waste of taxpayer money. What this intruder did not know was this family had a terminally ill child. The parents had lost their jobs due to taking care of the child and turning to government funding was the only way to care for their daughter and her medical needs. This was to be their child's last birthday and they planned to celebrate it with a proper cake. The family did not disclose the circumstances to the judgmental person. They made a choice not to spend time excusing their behavior or explaining that the judgement placed on them was cruel. They went on to live their lives celebrating the time they had left with their daughter. Situations like this can be avoided if judgments and assumptions are not made and needs are recognized, rather than focusing on behavior.

There are many individuals who share openly that they have an autism diagnosis or choose to share in specific situations. They may do this to self-advocate, to reach out for support or accommodations, to share their personalities, to connect with other people, to explain some of their struggles, or to promote acceptance of variability or biodiversity. As more and more representations of ASD are seen in communities, there must be an understanding and respect for the many different people represented on the autism spectrum. Autism friendly professionals will allow the person or family to take the lead in disclosing and sharing about their autism. If they mention autism, acknowledge it. If they refer to themselves as having ASD or being autistic, do not ignore it. If they avoid the word, do not pressure them to talk about it. If they communicate they want to be referred to as autistic or if they prefer first person language – honor their preference. Listen to what they are saying. They will provide the information they are comfortable with and what is needed to guide the conversation.

Conceptualizing Autism

Often families must navigate the world of autism which can include processing through several topics that can be controversial or wide ranging in opinion. There are commonly strong differing views in the "autism community" on whether to focus on finding a cure for ASD, accepting and loving a person for who they are, or if this is logically the next generation in intelligence and advocating for neurodiversity. Treatment options are divided between medical, therapeutic, behavioral, holistic, and educational, with some opposing the term treatment and any reference to ASD being considered a disease or disorder. Some families refuse to join a side in these arguments and prefer to implement a more eclectic approach. These parents are guided by hoping for the best quality of life for their children while loving them every day for who they are. Some of the divisions in autism can become deeply passionate and sadly, some shaming of parents or autistic individuals can take place by other parents and autisitc individuals. Historically autism families have been seen as fighters, but as resources and information become more widely available, these families might better be described as warriors. Many families in the early awareness of autism paved the way for current families by battling to get education and awareness about ASD acknowledged and resources for their children implemented.

As resources and support organizations develop, there is a discussion of partial advocacy or partial representation. This concept is where one group or one person takes the position of speaking on behalf of the whole, when in actuality they represent only a subgroup of an entire population or community. Specifically speaking about the contention in the autism community, Lutz (2020) points out:

> But these battles really boil down to just one question: Who decides what's best for those who can't speak for themselves, the severely

autistic individuals who will require upwards of $2.4 million in care over the course of a lifetime? Should it be parents, professionals, or should it be autistic self-advocates?

To have one group speak for the entirety of the autism community can have significant consequences. A person who feels stifled in job promotion opportunities because of their use of literal communication has a completely different experience and needs than someone who is unable to cross the street by themselves or do any life function independently. For one group to take the position of spokesperson for all with ASD just because they hold the same diagnosis or an autism degree, could be a great disservice to families affected by ASD. This practice causes families and individuals to face either unachievable expectations or confining them to boundaries where progress should be limitless. This affects families by confusing and further dividing them. One group might advocate for less targeted services and more independence, while another group believes there are limited individualized services impacted by the pressure for full inclusion. Social media has become one area that highlights this growing concern in the autism community. While it can be a good place to connect with other families, it can also often expose families to negative platforms that promote contention or encourage choosing sides.

A Family's Story (The Walkers)

Background – The Walkers were married with a five-year-old neurotypical daughter when they had Max. At age five, Max was diagnosed with autism. The marriage between Brad and Sarah Walker was problematic at the time Max was diagnosed. Within a year of the diagnosis, the Walkers were divorced. The two children lived with their mother full-time and dad was supposed to have regular visitations, but he rarely participated. Sarah Walker was accepting of Max's diagnosis and was genuinely interested in acquiring services for her son. Brad Walker was not supportive of the diagnosis and doubted its authenticity. Despite Brad's complaints, Sarah managed to place Max in occupational therapy and play therapy. She was also able to obtain IEP services for him as he began kindergarten.

Struggle areas – Sarah Walker was essentially a single parent raising two children (one with autism). Brad Walker would contact the children periodically, usually on holidays, and often did not contribute to their care or financial needs. Sarah worked full-time and had challenges navigating appointments, school meetings, and attending to Max's needs. Max's autism manifestations were milder and thus he could do many things for himself. He had some behavior difficulties at home but mostly his behavior manifested as odd or quirky to those around him. Max's older sister (Lilly) was often put into a parenting role to help take care of Max, especially with Sarah working full- time and struggling to keep the family organized. The parentification of Lilly created its own challenges, as often Lilly did not want to be responsible for Max and felt like her own needs were being neglected.

Max had a great many school struggles – mostly with peer and teacher interactions. Social interactions in general were challenging for Max and created issues for the family with extended family members and any social outings they might attempt. Often Max's school viewed him as a behavior problem and not as a child with ASD. They would not approve him for occupational therapy services at school and would often communicate to his mother that discipline was the issue, not autism. Sarah often found herself dealing with high levels of stress due to the school's threats of expelling Max and constantly calling her at work to complain about Max's behavior or to request she come and pick him up from school.

Strengths – Sarah Walker was a focused and determined parent. She was committed to meeting the needs of her children and devoted a significant amount of time to understanding autism and making sure that Max received the services he needed. Sarah, Max, and Lilly were a loving family. They seemed to have a strong bond with each other and overall a commitment to helping each other. Although Lilly could become resentful of Max, she was a devoted sister and child and cared strongly about her family. Max himself was often a pleasant child and he displayed a great deal of resiliency. He was also successful academically. He often demonstrated high academic ability, which helped him with some of his school struggles.

Supports and services – Shortly after Max received his diagnosis of autism, his mother placed him in occupational therapy, play therapy, and obtained an IEP. Max was able to access the therapies he needed throughout his childhood. Occasionally, Sarah would implement additional services for Max and for the most part, his therapies were a great source of support for Max and the family. Additionally, Sarah's mother provided support for the family. She would often watch the children when Sarah had to work, she would take Max to appointments, provide financial support, and seemed to be insightful about Max's autism issues. Lilly was also able to participate in a siblings group for children who had a brother/sister with autism. She found this experience to be helpful and met other children who were dealing with some of the same issues. Lilly developed a couple of friendships from this group and maintained those friendships throughout her childhood. Unfortunately, outside of therapies and the maternal grandmother, the family did not receive much support. The father, other extended family members, and the community were not supportive and often presented challenges for the family.

Autism friendly experience – The Walker family could be described as representing what many families experience regarding autism friendliness. Some things worked well for the family, such as their therapies. They were fortunate to connect with professionals who understood autism and provided an ongoing autism friendly support for the family. Outside of their therapies, there existed many people and situations that were not autism friendly. Max's school provided little understanding to the family and regularly brought more stress onto the family. Community endeavors were often not welcoming. The family regularly experienced negative reactions from store clerks, church staff, and the general observing public. For the Walkers, their autism friendly experience was a manifestation of the positive and the negative that so many families encounter.

Grant (2020) put forth that ASD is a systemic issue that affects the identified child and the whole family system. Parents and other family members are greatly involved in the experience of autism when a child in the family receives the diagnosis. Parents often must develop new ways of navigating and managing their family, adapting to a condition for which they had neither planned nor prepared. The hardest parts of autism are certainly the struggles which can be significant. But struggles are not all that exist in an autism family. Families with an autistic child can present in ways and enjoy life like any other family. Love abounds and often great unconditional love and support. Forgiveness is frequent. Joy comes from the simplest of things and the simplest things are often treasured and appreciated. There are always new things to discover and success is measured in centimeters rather than meters. Clay McGranahan (an autistic adult) communicated, "Autism redefines success. What you once expected to gauge your success and accomplishments by changes as you grow in your experience with autism" (C. McGranahan, personal communication June 6, 2010). This change in recognizing small and redefined achievements is what moves families affected by ASD forward on this incredible and unprecedented journey.

5 Autism and Communities

Marshall (2019) contended that for those with ASD, community engagement is often the end goal; that measure of success for which autistic individuals, their families, and professionals all strive. Increased and ongoing participation in one's community can have a positive impact on social competence and quality of life. Professionals experience satisfaction when individuals with autism reach identified communication or social goals and when families appear "ready" to take on the challenge and prepare for family "trips into the community." However, in spite of all that positive momentum, autistic individuals and families often report upsetting or disappointing community experiences. Long wait times at restaurants resulting in "meltdowns." Judgmental looks or comments from grocery store shoppers. A haircut that ends before the scissors actually cut any hair. Being asked to leave a church service. Feelings of embarrassment, anger, defeat, and the longing for a more accepting community.

Looking out from the bubble of ASD, there can be hope in improving community participation and success. Those differently abled who are actively working and living in neurotypical communities can fathom the idea that full inclusion is near. Over the years, attitudes have changed, people are accepting, and accommodations are being made. When a person is surrounded by compatible people working toward the common goal of community inclusion, it draws other like-minded people, and those people expand and continue the spread of positive impact. There is an increase in newsfeeds, stories, and conversations about the movements, efforts, and successes of autistic individuals within communities and the nation. There is much to feel positive about. However, many individuals with autism, once out of the bubble and in the day-to-day real world, continue to experience the feelings of being an outsider.

Individual communities, news stories, and social media highlight the differently abled prom kings and musical prodigies who are undoubtedly worthy of accolades. Occasionally there is a message of acceptance or feel-good event targeting inclusion. But, until the family affected by ASD no longer feels singled out and the prom royalty is won and highlighted with an ASD diagnosis portrayed with a sense of normalcy, and no ableism

DOI: 10.4324/9781003105633-6

attached, there will still be community struggles and separation. ASD should not be considered a taboo, untouchable, or a novelty subject. It is important to present information authentically and embrace the connections that develop naturally among those who are curious and willing to learn about others and who they are as an autistic person.

Families often have a challenge with community integration because of media portrayals of what autism looks like. Movies, characters, and television programs can sometimes present important depictions of ASD, which helps promote awareness, acceptance, and interest. Unfortunately, many of these presentations are fictional and struggle to adequately present the full view of the autism spectrum. The media is the first point of knowledge of ASD for many people, whether it is highlighting a missing child or showcasing a character in a major motion picture. Arguably, autism awareness is much more present in our society than 25 years ago, but struggles remain. A family shared a story of planning a move to another state and contacted that state's Chamber of Commerce to ask about autism resources. A week later they received a mailing envelope full of abuse pamphlets. The community was terribly unaware of autism. Most people today will have heard the word autism and have some type of thought about it, but will lack accurate depictions of autism. Often for communities it is an issue of resources and education. Do the community members know anyone who has ASD, and/or do they know where to access information and resources?

Often there remains a lack of understanding of autism unless it somehow touches a person's life, and they can experience a person behind the diagnosis. Autism is becoming more present in everyday life in both a personal and professional context. Some communities are embracing autism awareness and taking it to the next level of community integration. There are many positives that come from ASD awareness campaigns. Some examples include businesses asking to be trained about employment accommodations for those with ASD. Museums, restaurants, theaters, and other venues are hosting sensory safe and autism friendly events. Schools are advocating for inclusion and equality in educational experiences. There is a great deal to do before the autism bubble is removed and full community coexisting is in place, but the journey is showing to be effective.

Integration, Inclusion, and Culture

ASD can often be an invisible diagnosis, especially for those with a mild impairment. It may be first recognized by behavior. The community must decide not to judge but decode the behavior to determine how to proceed with inclusion and acceptance. Looking toward the future, autisitc people are no longer staying home. They are active in schools and their communities. A new generation of peers are growing up alongside those with autism. These people will be their future coworkers, their bosses, and their friends, building communities together. Inclusion is defined as the practice or policy of including and integrating all people and groups in activities, organizations, political processes, etc., especially those who are disadvantaged, have suffered discrimination, or are living with disabilities. Communities are embracing inclusion efforts because people with disabilities have rights and can be valuable members of the community. Those with autism have a right to access, right to services and goods, accommodations, and a right to offer their skills and insights to better the community.

As a community and its members become educated about ASD and begin to understand inclusion efforts, there is a risk of generalization. This is similar to what happens with media portrayals of autism. Not everyone with ASD is the same. It is important that the whole spectrum is completely and explicitly part of the conversation. Businesses and organizations within a community must understand that not all autistic people need the same type or level of support. While creating inclusive situations there is risk of over-reaching support for those who do not want help or prefer that their diagnosis does not become their identity. Inclusion efforts must be intertwined with neurodiversity awareness. There must be a willingness to provide support and accommodations that is buttressed with listening to the individual and/or family affected by ASD and letting them be the lead voice in what they need and do not need.

Communities are also impacted by law as it pertains to those with ASD and related conditions. In 1990 the Americans with Disabilities Act (ADA) became law. This civil rights law prohibits discrimination against people with disabilities. The law exists to ensure that people with disabilities have the same rights and opportunities as others. Findings of the law include:

1. Physical or mental disabilities in no way diminish a person's right to fully participate in all aspects of society, yet many people with physical or mental disabilities have been precluded from doing so because of discrimination; others who have a record of a disability or are regarded as having a disability also have been subjected to discrimination.
2. Historically, society has tended to isolate and segregate individuals with disabilities, and, despite some improvements, such forms of discrimination against individuals with disabilities continue to be a serious and pervasive social problem.
3. Discrimination against individuals with disabilities persists in such critical areas as employment, housing, public accommodations, education, transportation, communication, recreation, institutionalization, health services, voting, and access to public services.
4. Unlike individuals who have experienced discrimination on the basis of race, color, sex, national origin, religion, or age, individuals who have experienced discrimination on the basis of disability have often had no legal recourse to address such discrimination.

5. Individuals with disabilities continually encounter various forms of discrimination, including outright intentional exclusion, the discriminatory effects of architectural, transportation, and communication barriers, overprotective rules and policies, failure to make modifications to existing facilities and practices, exclusionary qualification standards and criteria, segregation, and relegation to lesser services, programs, activities, benefits, jobs, or other opportunities.
6. Census data, national polls, and other studies have documented that people with disabilities, as a group, occupy an inferior status in our society, and are severely disadvantaged socially, vocationally, economically, and educationally.
7. The nation's proper goals regarding individuals with disabilities are to assure equality of opportunity, full participation, independent living, and economic self-sufficiency for such individuals.
8. The continuing existence of unfair and unnecessary discrimination and prejudice denies people with disabilities the opportunity to compete on an equal basis and to pursue those opportunities for which our free society is justifiably famous, and costs the United States billions of dollars in unnecessary expenses resulting from dependency and nonproductivity.

The ADA is one of America's most comprehensive pieces of civil rights legislation that prohibits discrimination and guarantees that people with disabilities have the same opportunities as everyone else to participate in the mainstream of American life – to enjoy employment opportunities, to purchase goods and services, and to participate in state and local government programs and services. Its purposes include:

1. To provide a clear and comprehensive national mandate for the elimination of discrimination against individuals with disabilities.
2. To provide clear, strong, consistent, enforceable standards addressing discrimination against individuals with disabilities.
3. To ensure that the federal government plays a central role in enforcing the standards established on behalf of individuals with disabilities.
4. To invoke the sweep of congressional authority, including the power to enforce the fourteenth amendment and to regulate commerce, in order to address the major areas of discrimination faced day-to-day by people with disabilities.

Arguably, nothing compares to the Americans with Disabilities Act (ADA) in terms of helping those with autism and other disorders/disabilities gain valued presence in communities. Unfortunately, many individuals with autism must access this law in order to be treated fairly and given the same opportunities as neurotypical individuals. Community stories abound with issues of discrimination, stigmatization, and prejudice against those with autism and other disabilities. Part of being autism friendly means being aware of the laws that dictate rights to those with autism and committing to abiding by those laws. For more information on the ADA visit www.ada.gov.

Autism has long existed as a subculture within a greater cultural community. The autism community has promoted and utilized the terms neurotypical and neurodiversity to differentiate a different way of thinking, processing, and responding that is not less but different, not a problem, but an asset. The autism community is continually striving to be recognized for their unique composition, their efforts to collect important data regarding autism, and the gathering and articulation of ample resources that are useful. Many children who were diagnosed in the early 1990s are now adults and are speaking out and advocating for their rights and acceptance in ways that have not been seen before. Their advocacy efforts are having an impact on the recognition and understanding of the subculture of autism and how it is beginning to contribute to and change the understanding, sensitivity, and responses of the larger community (Grant, in press).

Autism affects people of all backgrounds, shapes, sizes, cultures and heritages. Different cultural factors can change how individuals experience autism in community life, influencing their interactions with family, schools, and health services. Cultural factors can also impact how autism is understood, interpreted, and accepted in different communities. Cultural myths about autism and other disabilities can deter people from seeking help. Information that may be useful for one person might be too much, or too little, or even confusing for another. There can even be many cultural differences within the same ethnic group, due to factors like country of birth and number of years in the United States. Research shows that in communities like Los Angeles, non-white families or recent immigrant families can have a more difficult time getting developmental services, which often delays a proper diagnosis (Children's Hospital Los Angeles, 2014). It is helpful for autism friendly communities to consider the following cultural considerations.

- Language
- Geographic location
- Religion
- Nationality
- Economic status
- Gender
- Beliefs and values
- Family structure
- Ethnicity

There is work that must be done to make the leap from rejection and isolation to integration and inclusion. Some of the barriers that stifle progress include the need for an active understanding of ASD and education and training to understand what integration and inclusion mean. Addressing fear, forced inclusion, stigmatization, and lack of employment supports are also pressing needs. Fortunately, there are many resources available for communities to learn about autism. It is important for communities wanting to increase their knowledge about ASD to find reputable sources. There are many national organizations as well as local nonprofits that provide information about autism. As a person studies ASD they must be careful not to get information from companies or influences that claim they can cure autism or that provide misleading and out of date information.

As communities gain knowledge about ASD through multiple reliable sources, they will begin to hear consistency of information, which is a good way to validate the information is accurate. There are many ways to approach learning and training about ASD, but there are core facts that will not vary. Looking toward field experts like Dr. Temple Grandin and Dr. Stephen Mark Shore and established organizations such as the Autism Society of America will remove the chance of getting misinformation. The *Autism Friendly Training Program* highlighted in this book references several reliable and valid individuals and organizations which provide accurate information about autism.

Communication and Social Awareness

As welcoming as a person, business, or organization might try to be, there are some natural and integral barriers built into navigating a community for an autistic person. No matter how perfectly planned an event is or thoughtfully arranged accommodations are, there is always the chance that something will go wrong, or expectations will not be met. For a person with autism, when things are different than expected or things change from what they have prepared for, it disrupts their dependence on predictability. This can leave the person feeling upset, confused, and vulnerable. Navigating the complexities of being a full and active member of a community can be challenging, especially without proper social and relational skills.

Many autistic people, both children and adults, prepare or practice for things in their lives. This may include studying social skills, reading social stories, or strategizing sensory aids. When someone leaves the security and familiarity of their home and ventures from their social circles there are social expectations that a person with autism may not naturally be able to understand, recognize, or utilize. There are many social affirming therapies and education styles a person with ASD may practice to learn basic to complex social skills. One of the most popular is Social Stories[TM] developed by Gray (2020). Dr. Linda Barboa (Obrey & Barboa, 2015) introduced PrepChats© in *Tic Toc Autism Clock*. PrepChats© are short conversations to help prepare a person for an event soon to follow that helps to create a sense of predictability and direction. Grant (2017a) developed a play-based protocol called *AutPlay® Therapy* to help children and adolescents learn and navigate social situations, and Grant & Turner-Bumberry (2020) developed *AutPlay® Therapy Play and Social Skill Groups* to help children develop social and relational skills.

As an autistic person ventures away from their home independently, they and their family have typically put in a significant amount of time and preparation to create a favorable experience. PrepChats©, Social Stories™, AutPlay® social skill groups, and predictability measures are all part of this effort to be as prepared as possible when venturing out into the greater community. Life is not always predictable, and this can be an ongoing challenge for those with ASD. Some individuals may struggle with interpreting their environment, social cues, and informal social "rules." Some will struggle to adapt and understand when things are different than expected, or something causes disarray in their schedule. These encounters can create fear, anxiety, avoidance, and behavior meltdowns.

Transitioning is a term used to describe leaving one life stage for another. One of the biggest life stage leaps is transitioning from high school to adult life. The community a student has known and relationships within that community can change drastically. If a person did not or could not learn to generalize social skills to fit the community experiences, this time can be a very anxious time. A person who is used to typing in a code to get lunch may need to learn to navigate a new payment system. So many little things that people generally pick up through environmental learning must be directly taught to a person with ASD and each new experience or change can be met with uncertainty and the need for support and acquiring of new knowledge.

If community members have a basic understanding of ASD (communication struggles plus sensory issues equals observed behaviors), they can better understand the autistic person and what they may be communicating. The goal of autism education and awareness is to decrease misunderstandings and better prepare communities to respond in an appropriate and helpful way if there is a communication, social, or sensory issue. Teaching people to distance themselves from the constraints of typical communication styles and unsaid rules can be important. For example, understanding non-typical language such as not being offended because someone with ASD says you smell funny. The word "funny" might mean something smelled different than what was expected to the autistic person. A person may not like it but that does not mean it is a bad or odorous smell and without proper autism awareness much can get misunderstood in social language. Another example might be a young person with ASD who cannot stand the smell of flowers and repeatedly says they stink because that is how to report something that is offensive to them.

Rejection, bullying, and being excluded are sadly a part of school and greater community environments. Autistic students from ages 8–17 years-old reported to researchers being bullied at a rate three times greater than their peers (StopBullying.gov, 2020). Hoover (2015) reported that bullying estimates vary depending on time-frames and reporters but by all reports, children with ASD are bullied more often than peers with other disabilities and more often than non-disabled peers, those with intellectual disabilities alone, and their typically developing siblings. One estimate summarizing data from a variety of studies indicates that broad-scale parent and children surveys report 44–77 % of ASD children being bullied within a one-month period, as compared to a rate of 2–17 % in self-report surveys of typically developing children. Another estimate based on a large parent survey suggests that as many as 94 % of autistic children and nonverbal learning disorders are bullied at some point in the past year as rated by mothers. Bullying experiences are basically negative/abusive social experiences which manifest in school and any peer meeting places around a community. Bullying can exist for a variety of reasons, including diminished ability to navigate the social system of their schools and community events, communication difficulties, their response to peer interaction, obvious signs of vulnerability, compromised self-regulation, or their response to their sensory environment.

Communities largely consist of social experiences. Some of these experiences are more formal and some are more friendly. Regardless, for the individual with ASD, each day and each event can be a challenge to navigate. The constant focus and consistent bombardment of communication and social navigation can develop other struggles. Anxiety, depression, and low self-worth can develop from not understanding social expectations and boundaries and the rejection that often comes from these interactions. These are barriers that can impact the autistic individual's experiences and growth. Our current climate is making shifts and beginning to recognize the need to provide a community atmosphere in which those with ASD can be comfortable and feel welcome. This is great progress toward not only integration and inclusion but supporting positive mental health for those with autism.

Sensory Awareness

Sensory overload can be a daily struggle for autistic individuals. They are usually at risk each time they leave their home and venture out into the community. Sensory friendly events are becoming more common as communities are recognizing this need and working to be more accommodating. Businesses are developing sensory friendly times where those with sensory issues can shop and eat as accommodations are made to minimize their sensory struggles. A benefit of sensory safe accommodations is that a sensory sensitive person can attend scheduled community events with the idea the exposures may help them to desensitize or develop coping mechanisms in a safe and accepting setting. This is accomplished by creating confidence so the individual can feel comfortable and make further efforts to attend or visit establishments during regular non-sensory friendly operations.

In addition to addressing sensory needs, many businesses and organizations are also addressing communication and ASD specific needs and barriers. Training is critical in helping businesses in communities become autism friendly. Through trainings like the *Autism Friendly Training Program*, communication barriers are addressed; from how to communicate with an ASD person who is nonverbal to those who are verbal and very literal. Training includes teaching staff and employees to address the person (not their caregiver), to avoid having a conversation about the person without including them, and how to be empathetic with social communication struggles. Training also includes a general understanding of ASD, which creates an ease and comfort level for all involved.

In the *Autism Friendly Training Program*, attendees learn to interpret behaviors they witness from those with ASD. What is a meltdown? What does predictability mean for a person with autism? What is stimming? How can an observer know whether the autistic person is comfortable and enjoying the experience or venue? Training also helps an employee recognize people who might be on the autism spectrum so support can be offered if necessary. A mother reported attending one of the largest local attractions in their town with her autistic son. The business had participated in many *Autism Friendly Trainings*. It was a big step for this mother to take her adult son alone to the venue. All was going well until his sensory limit was reached; the young man began to have a meltdown. What could have been a devastating experience ending in the police being called for support, ended quite differently than many past meltdowns the mother and son had experienced. During the dysregulated meltdown, the employees kept the flow of traffic going, giving the family space and time to move from the venue; never intervening, but never leaving them alone. The staff brought the family's belongings and walked an appropriate distance from mother and son. The employees smiled and made it known they were there if needed. The mother expressed her relief and pleasure at the way the business handled the situation and commented that instead of leaving defeated, the family could not wait to return another day to try again.

Sensory overload can be a threat to someone successfully navigating their environment. Informed community members learn to recognize a person addressing their sensory needs. They may see an individual wearing noise cancelling headphones, sunglasses or colored lenses, multiple layers of clothing, or hoodies. This is just a sampling of the variety of different supports or accommodations. It is important to remember the use of these items is not an invitation to ask questions about someone's personal needs.

A discussion of ASD is not off limits, but the individual or family should be the one to open the conversation. When approaching someone wearing sunglasses inside, do not engage in a conversation of why the person needs glasses. Instead, comment on how good the glasses look or inquire about where they were purchased. Let the conversation develop naturally for the individual to discuss their sensory issues.

Efforts to create sensory safe and autism friendly environments allow families affected by ASD to experience and enjoy their community. When sensory struggles or ASD compromise a successful and enjoyable night out, families will often divide. This division splits family time apart; they cannot participate in activities together. One example might be a game zone which may be too noisy for someone with auditory sensitivities to enjoy and participate. They may move quickly from game to game, attempting to play but not finishing, which makes it a hectic and expensive outing for the family. These circumstances cause the family to leave early or divide into groups to manage the situation, thus lessening their ability to be in the community enjoying their experience as a family.

Establishing a Sensory Friendly Event

The following is an example of how a sensory friendly event for autistic individuals and those with related conditions was created at a pizza place that had an accompanying game room. After hosting a special event for some young adults with developmental disabilities, the manager of the pizza place wanted to do something more for this population. The manager requested a meeting with ASD and sensory friendly trainers in the community to develop a plan.

From that meeting came intense sensory and ASD learning sessions for employees of the pizza place, including hands-on training. A complete sensory assessment of the game room (which included a racetrack, trampoline park, theater and laser tag, arcade games, and bumper cars) was commissioned. Adjustments were made to sound levels, flashing lights were turned off or covered, loud zones were identified, and noise cancelling headphones were provided. The 4-D theater provided options of having the moving seats on or off, lights turned up, and the sound turned down.

Discussions about additional issues ensued. A big concern was the expense for families to attend. An autistic person is likely to go from game to game within seconds of starting one, creating a situation where families were spending a lot of money with little time spent on game play. Families are often on tight budgets because of factors due to expenses related to caring for a child with autism and they needed a more cost-effective experience at the pizza place. The business decided they would charge a very minimal price for an unlimited game card. This was not their typical procedure but one they would implement for the needs of their autism customers.

The business wanted to create a special event/time when families affected by ASD, sensory issues, and related conditions could attend with the modified processes. It was decided to have the event one Saturday each month. This way families did not have to worry about missing an occasional event and it decreased the pressure of making the most of one day. Families were relieved of the pressure of feeling that this one day had to be successful. They could also leave if they felt it was the best choice, knowing they could return the next month. The business and the trainers wanted families to enjoy the venue and possibly progress to the point where they could feel comfortable attending during regular business hours without modifications.

Employee training for the pizza place included how to talk to customers and their families, how to use autism language the family preferred, how to approach a child or young adult with ASD, and what to do in case of a behavior meltdown. Employees wore special shirts so they were easily identified. During the last training just days before the launch of their new program, many of the workers reported feeling extremely nervous. After the first event, all employees were overjoyed at the success and loved meeting the families.

Families have continued attending these Saturday events at the pizza place years later. Grandparents, cousins, and friends now all join in. This was one of the first efforts at such a grand scale that led the way in this particular community for many other entertainment-based businesses to follow. While it is not the main goal of autism friendly events, there is often a financial benefit with increased sales and amazing reviews from families. When autism families find businesses that work toward servicing or accommodating all with inclusion efforts, they are loyal, supportive, and often very vocal – spreading the word to encourage patronage.

Kristen Gossett, *Beauty with some Extra Care: The Salon Experience*

Kristen Gossett owns and operates Extra Care Hair Co. located in a midsized city in the Midwest. In her story *Beauty with some Extra Care: The Salon Experience* she shares her experience of being a business owner in her community and dedicating herself to the process of being autism friendly to autistic clients and those with differing abilities.

> My passion as a stylist is to help my clients of all abilities look and feel their best. No matter what the needs are of any client, each person has their own unique challenges to navigate. A good stylist will take the time to understand these needs and ensure a positive experience. Prior to starting my own business, I worked in a chain salon designed solely around the needs of neurotypical clients and getting them in and out of the door as quickly as possible. The atmosphere

cosmetology schools prepare stylists for is a fast-paced, noisy, and rushed. As I sharpened my haircutting techniques, I felt the client-experience was lacking and the human connection lost in this salon culture.

During my time in this salon, a 14-year-old boy on the spectrum and his father came in to get a routine haircut, but there was nothing routine about serving the needs of this family. This child had stitches in his scalp from a recent surgery and other stylists refused to serve him because he required the use of incontinence protection and his body odor was very noticeable. The boy's father shared his feelings of dread about his previous experiences and hoped for his son to have the chance to gain confidence with a new haircut and not be retraumatized by the salon experience.

The sounds of the television, chatter, and overbearing music in addition to fragrances filled the room as he took a seat in my chair. I recognized this haircut needed to go at his pace. I took a deep breath, allowed myself to feel calm, and asked his permission to put the salon cape around his neck. I talked to my guest calmly throughout the haircut as I made each step of the process clear and predictable. He willingly sat in my chair throughout the entire haircut and when finished, looked at himself in the mirror with a satisfied expression. It was clear he was not just proud of his new look, but of his ability to successfully sit through his haircut as well.

I left work that night with a new feeling – like I had truly helped this family, and from this experience the idea for my business, Extra Care Hair Co. was born. In my salon, guests get the entire studio to themselves for #fearfreehaircare. I have scent-free products, quiet tools, dimmable lights, no music, an iPad for distraction, and kids' favorite – a prize box for being brave during the visit. Each of my guests have a free consultation appointment to come to the salon to experience feeling safe and comfortable before their visit as I hear about how I can accommodate their wishes. My person-first approach has evolved through researching best practices to serve my clientele. I have come to learn the unique needs of each person that sits in my chair. I keep detailed notes on each of my client's preferences, so their return visits can be even more successful. Since creating my business in April 2019, hundreds of people in my community have been grateful to find an alternative to the typical salon, and now, over 80% of my clientele are neurodivergent.

I have heard so many stories of traumatic experiences in salons from the families that find my business. The beauty industry does not equip stylists to serve people with sensory processing disorders, and it is a disservice to this community to not have trained professionals. After in-depth research and utilizing a strong community network in my hometown, I have been able to create a space where my guests can feel secure as they are served in an autism safe environment. I am able to provide specialized care for each of my clients with a calm, relaxing, and inclusive environment as the strong baseline for an enjoyable visit. My repeat customers become more confident in the salon chair as we build trust through routine, predictability, and consistency.

It puts a huge smile on my face to see my guest enjoying themselves, especially when it seemed like an impossible task in their previous salon visits. It reminds me exactly why I entered the beauty industry, to get the chance to take the time to see the inner beauty of each person and reflect these unique qualities in their outer beauty.

I created my salon to serve all kinds of people with all kinds of differences – for anyone who struggles in a world that does not recognize their unique gifts and appreciate their differences. I get to walk alongside my brave clients and hope this can be a reminder that there are dedicated, understanding helpers in the world that value uniqueness. Looking back on my time as a stylist, I am first and foremost proud of my clients and the successes they have had in my shop, no matter how big or small. I am, and always will be, a believer in the basic right to an inclusive environment. As a lover of ALL kinds of people, I see the beauty and value in everyone and get the honor of helping my clients and their communities see their inner beauty outwardly reflected through a little extra care.

Employment

Being autism friendly is not just about the interaction of the community with an autistic person and their families. It is also employment and the opportunities for people with a diagnosis to acquire pre-employment training, obtain and keep a job, receive accommodations, and develop relationships with coworkers. Being autism friendly will require businesses in any community to erase stigmatization around those with autism not being employable or only capable if menial jobs. As understanding of autism expands, businesses in the community can begin to recognize the employability of those with ASD.

According to the Centers for Disease Control and Prevention (CDC) (2020) employment information, there are higher rates for unemployment or under-employment for autistic teenagers and adults than for the population at large even though there are funded employment services and career development options for people diagnosed with autism. Although employers are attending workshops and trainings about employing someone with ASD and how to provide workplace accommodations, the CDC reports the reality being there are still many barriers to gainful employment. A greater number of children identified with ASD has led to a growing interest in the transition to adolescence and adulthood. For most young people, including those with ASD, adolescence and young adulthood are filled with new challenges, responsibilities, and opportunities. However, research suggests fewer young autistic people have the same opportunities as their peers without ASD.

Disability professionals can be shocked at the harsh reality of the job search for someone with autism. A job coach shared the experience of a client with autism who went to apply for a job at a local restaurant known for being current and trendy with fresh ideas. The job seeker was unable to leave their resume (the store would not accept it) and the person was rejected on the spot. The job coach was told by the store, "We don't hire people like that." The job seeker was not even given the opportunity to see if they were qualified or a good fit for the position. The issue and offense in this example displays a lack of professionalism and common courtesy that would have been extended to most neurotypical individuals in a similar position. As autistic people work toward employment or volunteerism they experience increased vulnerability as they put themselves in the position of looking for work or volunteer opportunities and often face rejection.

Carr (2017) reported that autistic adults may very well be the most disadvantaged disability group in the American workplace. Only 14 % of adults with autism held paid jobs in their communities. Yet only 2 % of all autism research funding goes to understanding adulthood and aging. While most research is focused on figuring out how to prevent or treat autism disorders when they are first diagnosed at young ages, we also have to remember that this work has not yet materialized as a solution for the more than 3.5 million Americans living with autism. The biggest hurdle in many instances seems to be helping them get to the point of being employees. Business can implement autism friendly measures by changing interview processes, where autistic individuals typically flounder. It can be helpful to allow a counselor to sit in on interviews, ensuring that someone familiar with autism participates in the interview. Many employers seem to agree that once an autistic worker lands a suitable job, they usually excel. Autism friendly change requires not only greater awareness but concrete alterations to the hiring and employee-support processes.

Research shows that there can be business benefits to hiring employees with autism. People on the spectrum often demonstrate trustworthiness, strong memories, reliability, adherence to rules and attention to detail. They are often good at coding (a skill that is in high demand), pattern recognition, strong attention to detail, and a very direct communication style. Beyond specific job skills, however, organizations increasingly recognize the importance of diversity to innovation. Neurodiversity, broadly defined as a diversity of thinking styles and abilities, is arguably especially important for innovative decision-making in the workplace (Oesch, 2019).

Employing autistic individuals means providing training to support their skills and training for the organization to create an inclusive workplace. For managers and coworkers, autism friendly awareness training can help them understand their colleagues with ASD and how to support them. Supervisors especially should receive training on effective communication strategies. Some businesses have implemented a buddy system where a neurotypical employee serves as a partner to the autistic employee providing them with support in navigating the workplace environment. More employers must strive to figure out a way to understand the skills of autistic people, implement autism friendly processes, and recognize the value in their efforts.

Communities and Safety

Another positive outcome from understanding ASD in the community is the increased safety for people with autism. There are now nationwide efforts to train first responders about autism. STARS for Autism and many national autism nonprofits have programs and information on first responder training including the *Autism Friendly Training* highlighted in this book. A large component of this training is how to communicate and listen to the families and caregivers in emergency situations. The family/ caregiver knows the person at risk the best and can provide critical information to the first responder. One family shared a story that their child, limited to only echolalia (meaningless repetition of another person's spoken words, repetition of speech by a child learning to talk), was a flight risk, which often caused the family great distress. The family learned that when he went missing, they should first check the neighbor's pool, then begin an extended search. Through trial and error, they came up with a foolproof plan. Whoever was looking would walk around and repeat, "Here I am," quickly receiving an echo back of "Here I am." No other call or plea would get a response from the child. Only someone close to the child would be able to give that insight which would be valuable information for first responders trying to locate this child.

Many actions that trigger suspicion from a first responder are common autistic behaviors, from not responding to questions, wearing concealing clothing, and lack of eye contact. A young adult male reported to his therapist that he had an encounter with a police officer. The young adult was driving down a road and was pulled over by a police officer. The police officer had pulled him over due to his car matching the description of a car they had been looking for. The young adult with ASD did not navigate the social interaction with the police officer well. He did not make eye contact, had to take time to process the questions that were being asked by the officer, and to the officer, the young adult just didn't seem to be acting "normal." The officer thought the young adult was on drugs and took him to the police station for further testing. The young adult had not committed any crime, was not taking drugs, and was terribly upset by the situation. The police officer made several negative assumptions about what were, in actuality, autism behaviors. The result was creating a traumatic experience for a young autistic adult.

By looking at a situation with the assumption that it could be autism, the approach and perhaps the outcome could change. Vital information in *Autism Friendly Trainings* is essential as increased numbers of families and autistic individuals are navigating their community and encountering various first responders. There are numerous positive outcomes in communities, from awareness to inclusion efforts, but much is still lacking. One striking oversight is that autism is not always included in first responders' professional training or development. As inclusion and independence are increasing at a rapid rate, there are improvements that need to be implemented in order to keep first responder training commensurate with autism needs. With greater community involvement, the risk of altercation increases exponentially, and it is vital to equip first responders with strategies and information.

As community openness increases for those with ASD, the topic of wandering and elopement is essential to cover when learning about autism. The more the public knows about this risk, the more supportive they can be to the person with autism and their loved ones. Wandering, also referred to as eloping, is characterized by an autistic person leaving a known location, or leaving the care of the person supporting them, and proceeding unsupervised. The terms refer to an individual with cognitive challenges or special needs who wanders, runs away from, or otherwise leaves a caregiving facility or environment. The National Autism Association (2012) reported caregiver challenges concerning elopement behavior.

- Wandering, also referred to as elopement, was ranked among the most stressful ASD behaviors by 58% of parents of elopers.
- 62% of families with children who elope were prevented from attending/enjoying activities outside the home due to fear of their child wandering.
- 40% of parents have suffered sleep disruption due to fear of elopement.

A study in 2012 conducted by the Interactive Autism Network, found that nearly half of children with autism spectrum disorder (ASD) at some point attempt to wander or bolt from a safe place. Using parent surveys, the researchers studied over 1,100 autistic children ages 4–11 years. They found that these children demonstrated much higher instances of wandering than their neurotypical siblings. By increasing awareness of this behavior and the risks to an unsupervised person who is dependent on family members and caregivers, those impacted by ASD are more likely to enjoy their communities with increased confidence and decreased stress.

Communities can implement autism friendly principles by being aware of elopement challenges and assisting families in preventative and support measures. Some strategies include developing a safety plan with neighbors, schools, and community members, providing identification jewelry (such as bracelets or necklace charms) for children to wear, designing and providing wearable technology with built-in GPS systems, and utilizing amber alert systems so individuals in the community can be helpful in finding children who are missing. Increased community awareness and education can help tremendously in the case of elopement issues and are an essential component of being an autism friendly community.

Places of Worship and Social Gatherings

Many communities throughout the world have made great strides regarding integration and inclusion. Entire cities are taking steps and declaring themselves autism friendly. One adverse consequence is that familiarity breeds self-declared experts. There are those who will give advice to families without regard to the families' efforts, ideas, experiences, or beliefs. This advice can make the family feel judged or uncomfortable. It can cause a family to feel they are in a spotlight of ongoing assessment as others freely comment on their loved one and their behaviors. This familiarity can also cause comparisons. They may compare someone with autism to a person that has been seen in a newsfeed story. Comparisons range from "Why isn't your child able to do this?" to "Look, you don't have it that bad."

One family reported feeling uncomfortable with comparisons at their church. They felt they were always being watched, but rarely approached. Staring eyes were part of Sunday service for this family. While this family was focused and did not let it deter them from church attendance, it was uncomfortable. It became increasingly hard to engage in conversations. Then, one Sunday, the mother sat in the foyer with her wiggling child. Another woman joined her and said she was glad to be able to see them up close. Not sure what that meant, the mother patiently waited. The conversation continued, "There are a few of us that compete to sit behind you because we love watching your children and how you interact with them. It is the best part of the service." This conversation continued and was luckily a welcoming and positive one for the mother. It also became a turning point for the mother and her family to feel more accepted in their church. At times, it is difficult for families to know if they are being judged or not; it is easy to assume that others are being judgmental when speaking about autism, as that is often the case. Church and places of worship can be a complicated challenge for anyone with ASD considerations. It can feel welcoming and warm or it can be closed off and rejecting. Many families have reported terrible stories of judgment and rejection they have received from churches. Some families report they have given up trying to attend church as they have had so many negative experiences. Barboa and Allen (2018) postulated:

As members of the disability community, many stories and situations tug at our heartstrings. This is never truer than when we hear the pain in the voices of parents as they tell of being rejected in churches because they have a disabled family member. We hear the same scenarios day after day as we listen to parents tell of failed attempts to attend church. Some are frantically searching for a solution. Others have given up and no longer even try to take the family to church. It is important for families facing the enormous challenge of raising special needs children to find religious support and have the spiritual edification they seek. They want this for themselves and they need it for their children.

A church or any place of worship is only one place autistic people and their families struggle in their community. Social organizations, clubs, extracurricular activities, community events, etc. all hold the possibility of success or rejection for families affected by ASD. Places, situations, or times where there is increased risk of a negative outcome can include any event or activity, but most significantly school settings, employment, social events, and relational meetings. All of these areas have the potential for bullying/victimization, unpredictability, sensory overload, dangerous or potentially dangerous environments, and false assumptions. Basically, anytime the person with autism ventures outside their home into the greater community there is risk.

Becoming educated about and supporting autistic individuals is not a onetime accomplishment. There are constantly new things to address and learn and there are consistently new families and individuals to assist. Showing patience and understanding for families who are learning how to best support their autistic child or for autistic people struggling with navigating their community is always a welcomed approach. One of the best ways for communities to grow toward being inclusive, autism friendly, and welcoming is to dedicate themselves not to a onetime training but to a community lifestyle commitment of awareness and support.

A Community's Story

Background – Jimmy lived with his two parents and older brother. They lived in the same small community his entire life. Jimmy had autism, a chromosome disorder, and co-occurring medical conditions. His impairments were such that he required continuous care and was unable to live independently. Jimmy spent his young years in special education settings and special schools focused on working with children with his issues. He also participated in various therapies and interventions mostly designed to help improve his skill deficits. Due to his medical conditions, Jimmy was occasionally on a feeding tube, needing to wear a helmet, or needing to use a wheelchair. He received constant support from his parents, extended family members, and in-home support workers.

Struggle areas – Like most families affected by autism and related conditions, Jimmy and his family struggled to find educational placements in their community that could meet Jimmy's needs. The local school district was not helpful and often devaluing of Jimmy and his family. The family eventually had to transport Jimmy to a larger city to gain proper educational supports. They also struggled to find professionals to work with Jimmy, including speech, occupational therapy, and mental health services. Every professional service Jimmy required aside from his family doctor had to be accessed in another city. Jimmy's family spent a great deal of time traveling each week to acquire services. Community involvement was often a struggle as well. Due to Jimmy's impairments, he would often require special accommodations at events. The family experienced a great deal of negativity, often by others in the community expressing displeasure with the way Jimmy would be behaving and criticizing his parents.

Strengths – Jimmy benefited from not just immediate family support but extended family support as well. Jimmy's family spent most of his childhood living in the same house and this enabled the family to acquire several neighbors who knew the family well and often provided support. The family was able to find a local church that was open and willing to learn about Jimmy's issues and open to making accommodations and support the family and Jimmy in any way they could. The neighborhood and local church support were strengths for the family residing in this community and were often cited by the family as meaningful and critical to their success.

Jimmy had a strong interest in police people and police cars. His family was able to form a strong positive relationship with their local police force. All the police people knew Jimmy and treated him very favorably. He was allowed to have birthday parties at the police station and sometimes a police person would come by their home and let Jimmy sit in a police car. The positive relationship the family formed with the local police department was cited by the family as one of the primary strengths they saw in living in their community. The neighbors', church, and police response in this community also highlights how incredibly beneficial this type of community support can be for families and individuals affected by autism.

Supports and services – The supports and services that could be accessed in Jimmy's local community were limited. A great deal of this limitation was due to the size of the community and there simply not being services available. Jimmy's story highlights how community support is much more than access to professional services. Neighbors, churches, store managers, police, mail people, etc. all make up even the smallest of communities. Many of these individuals were invaluable to Jimmy and his family and each in their own way provided great support to his family. While most of Jimmy's professional services were accessed outside of his local community, he and his family experienced many supports from several of the people who shared space with them in their community.

Autism friendly experience – When Jimmy was ready to graduate from high school (which he had been attending in a special school for children with ASD), the family discovered the school did not have a graduation ceremony. Many of Jimmy's cousins had attended and graduated from the community public school and Jimmy had expressed that he wanted a graduation like the ones he had attended for his cousins. The family contacted the local public school to ask if Jimmy could participate in their graduation ceremony and the school told the family he could not participate. Upon hearing this, a neighbor and friend contacted his friend, who owned a nearby racetrack. Jimmy was fond of cars and the friend set up a graduation party for Jimmy at the racetrack. It was a large enough venue that many people could be invited, and Jimmy was thrilled. Another neighbor made a graduation sign for the family to place in their front yard and yet another arranged for Jimmy to ride in a race car onto the racetrack during his graduation party and another donated a graduation gown and cap for Jimmy to wear. The graduation party happened with many community members attending and celebrating Jimmy. It was truly a community affair and exemplified the power of community support focused together to be autism friendly.

The *Autism Friendly Training Program* highlighted in this book provides many tools to assist communities with being autism friendly – from guides to social stories to visuals to practical advice. Several strategies are given for professionals across businesses, organizations, and support services. Each business, organization, or agency creates a greater sense of community inclusion by becoming aware, sensory safe, and autism friendly. These efforts are leading the way to make inclusion training less of a distinct effort and more of an assumption that it is the norm to be friendly, sensitive, and accommodating to all. Community leaders will want to pay special attention to Chapter 9 of this book, which highlights the *Autism Friendly City Training Program.*

6   Being Autism Friendly

The ability to effect any purposeful change in a society or to implement an initiative on a large-scale basis is dependent upon participants having a clear understanding of both the target and the path suggested to achieve that paradigm. This is true as we set out to chart a course toward becoming an autism friendly society. Two of the cornerstones of such a goal would certainly be establishing a shared understanding of the terms used and mapping the most logical route to achieve the goal. This chapter highlights what it means to be autism friendly and serves as the introduction to the second half of this book, which is more pragmatic in describing the *Autism Friendly Training Program*.

Centuries ago, forward thinkers invented a tool which would revolutionize future generations – the map. As primitive maps evolved into the use of the modern Global Positioning System (GPS), their usefulness continued to rely on one basic cornerstone – knowing the destination. Even as sailors sought guidance from the map in the sky, a successful journey depended on defining markers such as the North Star and recognizing the intended target. In the same way, providing a clear definition of the term autism friendly is essential in bringing the concept to fruition. The most useful definition will serve as a guide in establishing both goals and expectations.

According to the International Board of Credentialing and Continuing Education (IBCCES) (2020), there are no set standards for meeting the designation of autism friendly. While this lack of clarity allows communities or businesses a large amount of freedom in making the declaration, this is also a problem. Entities at this point can merely declare themselves to be autism friendly with no real training or understanding. The IBCCES reported that of 1,000 parents surveyed, 97% stated they felt it was not meaningful for organizations to merely claim to be autism friendly. They reported the term often carried very little weight and was sometimes of doubtful credibility. To clearly establish universal goals and expectations, the designation must be clearly defined. Only then can it be an accepted and valued part of our vocabulary and discussion.

A review of the literature provides one definition that meets established requirements. Wikipedia (2020) defined autism friendly as:

DOI: 10.4324/9781003105633-7

being aware of social engagement and environmental factors affecting people on the autism spectrum, with modifications to communication methods and physical space to better suit individual's unique and special needs.

This definition requires an understanding and a flexibility in both interpersonal and public relationships.

Stebbins (2016) explained that the concept of autism friendly evolved as society began thinking differently about disabilities in general. At that point, society stopped thinking solely about how to change individuals with disabilities to better fit the environment. People began to realize that the environment should actually accommodate the unique needs of the individual. Educational institutions and communities began to understand that diversity does not demand exclusion. Rather, diverse people can thrive in a welcoming world. That accepting world will include adapting physical spaces, along with changing attitudes and mindsets that are understanding and accepting of differences.

A closer look at the concept of autism friendly through this lens brings us to the conclusion that this standard of behavior must be applicable to the full gamut of characteristics which define autism itself: struggles in communication, sensory issues, and social behavioral differences. The challenge inherent in this definition is to create an awareness of all factors affecting those with autism and develop ways to modify the environment and our own interactions in order to facilitate increased quality of life.

Sensory Awareness

To fully digest the definition proffered here, we must circle back to the basics of autism and revisit the impact that each of the senses may have on the individual. We must sharpen our ability to discern when a given sensory stimulus is causing a reaction due to being perceived as too strong or too minimal. The individual may be hyposensitive or hypersensitive in one or more of the senses (Grant, 2018b). The inconsistency of the sensitivity level adds to the difficulty. With this understanding, we can accommodate the person's needs through environmental modifications.

Obrey and Barboa (2015) detailed the chaotic ramifications of sensory sensitivities. Each of the senses must be understood in order to make any needed accommodations. Desensitization to the various sensory stimuli is complex. Most people are familiar with the five basic senses – vision, hearing, taste, touch, and smell. Fewer are well-versed in the additional senses of vestibular, proprioception, and interoception. To be autism friendly requires at least a basic understanding of sensory functioning and how an individual with autism can be affected,

A study by Enoch et al. (2019) reported empirical evidence that 88 % of people ranked sight as their most valued sense, followed by hearing. We gather a tremendous amount of information visually, but for those not processing it efficiently visual stimuli can be distressing. Some people are hypersensitive to light; they wear hats and sunglasses to avoid the pain caused by the light. On the other hand, some are driven to seek light and may cause themselves harm by staring at the sun or other bright lights. Multiple visual stimuli can actually cause a person to feel exhausted. Sensitivity to light is not the only effect of sensitivity to visual stimuli. Others may have difficulty shifting their gaze from one object to another. This is also the source of eye contact avoidance. An overlooked aspect of visual perception difficulty is the inability to tolerate visual movements. People or objects moving around in their field of vision cause extreme distress. These individuals may withdraw from group activities due to the visual stimuli of movement. They may even be afraid of seemingly innocuous visual movements, such as the sight of a butterfly or a fly. Another result of visual perception confusion is difficulty identifying the source of the stimuli.

Barboa and Bradshaw (2018) reported an anecdote by a mother wherein her young daughter kicked, screamed, bit, and ran from the doctor when he tried to use a small flashlight to look in her mouth. The girl mistakenly perceived the light as fire and thought the doctor was trying to put fire in her mouth. It is challenging for some autistic individuals to focus because their minds are constantly taking snapshots in milliseconds of things around them. Some parents have reported they believe this may be why their children with ASD have difficulty reading facial clues and maintaining eye contact (Barboa and Obrey 2017).

Enoch et. al. (2019) found that the second most highly valued sense is hearing. People rely heavily on the ability to not only hear, but to process hearing into meaning. A large amount of information is acquired through the auditory sense, also known as the sense of hearing. Auditory sensitivities can distort the incoming stimuli. The autistic person may perceive sounds as being much louder than they actually are, or they may seem to not notice the sounds. When people are subjected to sounds that are uncomfortable to them, this may result in unwanted behaviors. One such behavior may be an individual humming or producing a chanting sound. This may be an attempt to mask the noises that are bombarding their sensory system.

Just as each individual's sense of taste is different from another person's, this variation can be extreme in someone with ASD. The differences can be exaggerated to the point that acceptable foods are reduced to a very minimal list. Many parents express that their autistic children will only eat four different foods, rotating those foods from meal to meal. The individual's sense of taste can be highly distorted. Their confused sensory processing actually distorts their perception of foods they are tasting, causing the food to seem either tasteless or far too intense. The distorted gustatory sense, known as the sense of taste, might even result in the individual accidentally ingesting poisonous substances. Barboa and Luck (2017a) described a child who ate a strong, pungent onion every day for lunch, while refusing foods such as peaches, commonly enjoyed by children. Children with distorted taste preferences may also exhibit a condition known as pica. People who display pica have a compulsion to eat non-edible substances, such as paint chips or dirt. Understanding of the taste preferences and compulsions is needed when called upon to make environmental modifications in the area of taste.

Confused sensory processing of aromas may cause a fragrance to seem too strong or not noticeable at all. The sense of smell may need to be addressed if a modification needs to be implemented for an autism friendly environment. An autistic person may find the smell of flowers to be repulsive, while being drawn to noxious odors such as the exhaust from a bus. Others may be noted to be drawn to the smell of people's hair or body lotions. They may even be able to smell things that the neurotypical person cannot smell.

The same sensory processing confusions may apply to the sense of feeling and touch. This is the tactile sense. Often a person may describe a touch, especially a light touch, as being painful. Some may crave touch while others are repulsed by it. The feeling of the texture of clothing may be extremely irritating and cause behavioral meltdowns. The temperature of the room may cause strong reactions. Extreme sensitivity to temperature may cause them to want to disrobe. Understanding of the possible reactions is needed for an autism friendly environment.

In addition to those five commonly known senses, there are three which are lesser known. Vestibular, proprioception, and interoception abilities are also affected in people with ASD. Becoming autism friendly will require knowledge of these senses. The vestibular sense gives the mind information about where the body is in relation to the earth. It is a sense of balance and body movement. A possible result of vestibular confusion is a severe reaction of claustrophobia if the person finds themself in a crowd or in a small space. Children with vestibular challenges may avoid playground equipment that requires their feet to be off the ground. They may avoid fast moving activities, as those may be distressing to their sensory system. Conversely, they may be thrill seekers creating vestibular input because their bodies are not reading danger cues, such as height or speed.

Proprioception is the sensory system that provides feedback as to where a person's body is relative to the space surrounding them. Insufficient transmitting and processing of proprioceptive clues is seen as clumsiness, lack of coordination, and feeling challenged by sustaining movement patterns. The person may continually bump into objects and may display bruises. These children may be seen as playing too roughly with other children. Barboa and Luck (2017b) warned that parents of children who have proprioceptive issues are often reported to child protective services on the mistaken grounds of child abuse, due to the bruises visible on the child. The bruises are often caused by the child's clumsiness, falling, or even self-injurious behaviors.

Barboa and Luck (2017b) described the sense of interoception which refers to an individual's sense of what is happening within their body. As the body sends signals to the brain with messages such as hunger, sleepiness, pain, bathroom needs, nausea, and thirst, the sense of interoception is employed. People with autism may not receive these signals from the body in a typical way. They often have confusions about those signals that the body is sending to the brain. They may laugh or cry inappropriately, display eating or sleep disturbances, or have toileting confusions. Interoceptive sensations may be unreliable information for autistic individuals. When a neurotypical person feels hungry, that is a signal to eat. When they feel thirsty, their brain signals them to drink. When they feel tired, they recognize the feeling and they sleep. Barboa and Luck (2017b) reported research indicating people with ASD may actually have fewer neuroreceptors than others. They have trouble interpreting what their body is telling them. The person learning to be autism friendly will recognize the individual's efforts to avoid a certain sensation or to seek a certain sensation from the world around them and that the autistic individual may get erroneous signals from their own bodily receptors.

With the full range of senses being affected, professionals may be well advised to choose their battles and work through one irritant at a time. Vaughan (2014) stated that for some, sensory processing challenges will present as defiant behavior, opposition, or refusal to cooperate. These behaviors may develop out of a need to avoid or escape a challenging situation. When a person presents with sensory created behaviors, it is often the problematic behaviors that receive attention and the problematic behaviors that get addressed, while the root issue of the sensory challenge is ignored.

While a neurotypical person learns to employ coping strategies to deal with sensory exposures, an autistic person may be overwhelmed. This overload may result in unwanted behaviors. Expanding upon a list put forth by Obrey and Barboa (2015), overt behaviors that might signal possible sensory issues include:

- resistance or over-affinity to touch people or items,
- extremely picky about food (taste, shape, texture, smell, color, or other attributes),
- sensitivity to light or an obsessive attraction to light,
- avoiding eye contact or craving eye contact,
- craving or avoiding excessive movement,
- avoiding or fearing normal movement or moving obsessively,
- uninterested in new situations or seeks unique stimuli,
- may appear clumsy or misguided,
- easily distressed by unfamiliar or new things,
- over or under responsive to sounds/noises,

- inability to identify body signals such as hunger, tiredness, thirst, bathroom needs, and pain,
- and obsessive tendencies.

While the basic task in meeting the definition of autism friendly in the area of sensory sensitivities is to recognize the individual's needs and modify the environment accordingly, it is also necessary to be aware of competing sensitivities. One sense may overpower another (Obrey & Barboa, 2015). People may be dealing with competing senses continually throughout the day. The neurotypical person may watch TV and carry on a conversation at the same time, but the person with ASD may only be able to attend to one stimulus at a time. Obrey and Barboa further explained that both types of sensitivities (hypo and hyper) will most likely be present in each individual with autism. They suggested looking at individual traits when working or living with someone with sensory issues to better understand the person's individualized sensory challenges.

Everyone processes sensory information in differing ways. When our bodies process the incoming sensory stimuli, this is called sensory integration. We each tolerate different amounts of stimulation. Those individual variations in sensory tolerance are not a problem unless they begin to interfere with daily life activities (Barboa & Datema, 2016). Children and adolescents with sensory processing challenges may have struggles in most or all areas of their life. Along with sensory integration struggles, a person may also experience frustration, rejection from peers, academic struggles, self-esteem struggles, mislabeled and misunderstood behaviors, and emotional regulation challenges. Sensory processing challenges should be viewed as a spectrum of presentation. Each child or teen with sensory issues will be affected differently, with individual challenges and strengths (Grant, 2018b).

Communication Awareness

The same principles apply to detecting the communication struggles a person may be encountering. These challenges may stem from issues in expressing themselves or difficulties in understanding the communication from others. Upon determining the source of the communication struggle, modifications may be made to meet the individual's unique needs. The spectrum of language skills ranges from being nonverbal to advanced language abilities. The autism friendly person will be very aware that a nonverbal person may actually have good receptive language skills. Although they are not able to express themselves, they often understand what is being said around them. There are many ways in which a person may express themself, and a listener should honor the attempt in whatever form it is presented.

An autism friendly professional should be considerate of the communication struggles presented by any individual. Even a highly verbal autistic person may lack a "filter" when speaking. There is a tendency for those with autism to speak what is on their mind without any self-censoring. They may say what they think without understanding that the comment may be hurtful or inappropriate. The autism friendly person will not take offense if the individual makes an innocent comment about the listener's appearance. One example involves a speech-language pathologist ("Mr. Mike"), who took it in good humor when he was told, "Mr. Mike, you got dog teeth."

Another communicative characteristic that the autism friendly professional should be aware of is the tendency to repeat words, phrases, or paragraphs that the speaker has heard before. The listener will become familiar with the fact that even though words or sentences are coming out of the autistic person's mouth, they might not be meaningful functional communication, but rather just spoken words. The autistic person may recite single words, phrases, entire commercials, or movie scripts. The autism friendly professional will be aware that the individual may speak in a flat, monotone voice which may sound odd. The listener will make an effort to focus on what the person is saying rather than how it is being said.

There may be a wide spectrum of ability to construct sentences. The autistic individual may use some basic sign language, an electronic device, or may speak with an accelerated vocabulary. Listeners should be aware of confusions in the use of pronouns. For example, if a child is asked where their apple is, they may answer, "I ate her." Also, the autism friendly listener should not be surprised nor upset if the child with ASD refers to them as the opposite gender. Along with pronoun confusion, it is possible to hear difficulties in the use of prepositions. These are often ambiguous and difficult for this population to process. If a teacher tells a child to, "Put the book up now," the child may hold the book in the air, as they take the directive literally.

The neurotypical person uses a skill known as "code-switching" to adjust their vocabulary and tone of speech to the listener. The manner used to speak to friends at happy hour may differ strongly from the vocabulary and tone used when speaking to a boss. Neurotypical people speak differently to the school principal or the church pastor than to a brother at a family dinner. Autistic people might not understand the need for code switching. The person with autism may not adjust their speech to the listener. When talking to their friends and family they may sound like "the little professor," but may use inappropriately informal language at school (Barboa & Bradshaw, 2018).

Regarding receptive language, there is often a problem with understanding words that have multiple meanings. These are called polysemic words. The English language is abundant with these multiple-meaning words. In fact, it is difficult to think of a word in the English language that is *not* polysemic, other than words that are specific to a certain discipline or profession. Winchester (2011) documented 645 distinctly different meanings for the word "run" in its verb form alone. There are additional meanings if the noun form is included. For a person who is having difficulty processing two different meanings for a word, 645 is overwhelming. Further complicating the problem of polysemic words are the homophones in our daily speech. The word "bear," for example, is pronounced the same as the word "bare," and "whole" is pronounced the same as "hole." Understanding the English language can be demanding and confusing even for the neurotypical learner.

The same is true of idioms and figures of speech. Individuals with ASD tend to be literal thinkers and often do not understand idioms. A person who was told to, "Keep your eye on the ball," might ask how that would be possible. As they take things literally, they will have expectations based on the exact words spoken. If a customer with autism is told, "I'll be with you in a minute," they will expect help in less than 60 seconds. A good rule for the autism friendly person is to "say what you mean and mean what you say." Another area of difficulty that an autism friendly professional needs to be aware of is the difficulty with all-inclusive and generic words. Words such as "all," "none," "everybody," "class," "always," and "never" may be fairly meaningless to the autistic individual. They may not follow a directive such as, "Everyone stand by that wall," because they do not understand that the term "everyone" is all-inclusive and applies to them.

Behavior Awareness

Environmental or personal accommodations can increase quality of life in the area of social skills and behavior. By learning to identify precipitating factors, problems and meltdowns can be avoided or minimized. Keeping in mind that behaviors are a function of sensory issues and communication frustrations, the autism friendly person can often mitigate the behavioral challenges. The behaviors themselves are often the means by which a person is attempting to communicate. If a person lacks a functional form of communication, they will use behaviors to communicate their wants and needs (Grant, 2020). Barboa and Obrey (2017) suggested the autism friendly professional should be aware of common manifestations and behaviors an autistic individual may display such as:

- the need for predictability and a routine
- taking things literally,
- difficulty understanding sensory irritations,
- needing sensory stimulation,
- getting frustrated easily,
- constantly needing stimulation, calming, or alerting,
- misinterpreting things,

- lacking appropriate communication skills,
- exaggerating what they are actually feeling,
- difficulty with eye/face gaze,
- inability to interpret facial expression and other gestures,
- show little interest in others,
- may not understand humor,
- have an extreme attachment to a toy or other object,
- play with toys in unusual ways,
- fear things they need not fear, yet not being afraid of things they should fear,
- appear or really want to be alone,
- repeatedly do unusual actions,
- shun or crave physical contact with others,
- have outbursts due to sensory or communicative struggles,
- get upset if others are not following their perceived rules,
- lack appropriate response to pain,
- have difficulty self-regulating emotions,
- and have difficulty transitioning from one activity to another.

It is imperative to notice the direct relationship between sensory issues, communication processing/challenges, and behaviors. Each behavior is precipitated by sensory and/or communication frustrations and the behavior itself is a form of communication.

Through adopting a shared definition of the term autism friendly, an important step is taken in the journey toward realizing how to become autism friendly. The definition requires exploring possible ways to adjust communication methods and modify the physical environment to better suit the individual with ASD's unique needs. Barboa and Obrey (2017) urged those working autistic individuals to pay careful attention to the person's behavior; this is a guide to better awareness. Learning to understand and respect the individual's fears and discomforts is an important step on the journey to becoming autism friendly but this understanding is futile unless it precipitates change.

Sensory Processing and Environmental Awareness

Professionals should look closely at the response to various sensory stimuli and note that some of the responses result from people avoiding certain stimuli while others are seeking the stimulation. This dichotomy applies to all the sensory areas. To fully implement the autism friendly definition requires making some simple modifications to the environment and/or to communication processes which benefits all involved (Barboa & Datema, 2016). Prelock (2006) defined the environmental factors as those that are "outside or 'extrinsic to' the person and might include societal attitudes, cultural norms, laws, educational systems, and architectural considerations." Too often the term "environment" is understood as limited to the physical surroundings, but in reality, it encompasses much more. The environmental modifications mentioned in the definition pertain to the more wide-ranging systems, attitudes, and laws. These factors significantly broaden the scope of opportunities that are present for modifications.

Modifications to the environment may embody an extremely wide range, from minimal tweaks to large re-engineering of a system. Most will be small and easily implemented. Although each person with ASD is an individual and their needs will differ, we can look at suggestions that may meet the needs of many. Barboa and Luck (2017a) suggested thinking of each of the senses as two cups. Some people have an exceptionally large sensory cup and they seek continually to fill the cup and cannot seem to get enough stimuli. Other people feel they have an exceedingly small tolerance for sensory input, represented by a tiny cup, easily filled to overflowing.

Persons with visual sensitivities may manage much better if allowed to wear a cap or sunglasses, as they may be bothered by certain lights. Some may be dysregulated by rapid movements in their line of vision. A suggested modification would be to use gentle, slower, smoother movements. As rapid movements in their line of vision may be confusing to them, it will be helpful to explain the movements they see and help them adjust. Can they have a desk or workstation away from active movement? Can they wear their sunglasses in the classroom or office? Understanding the issues and allowing for accommodation/modification is what separates the autism friendly professional from the non-friendly professional.

If hearing sensitivities are noted, speaking in a calm voice can be helpful. Individuals may respond more to tone of voice than to exact words. One notable issue is the autistic person typically has difficulty filtering out background noise from the speech of someone talking to them. The voice of a person down the hall or in another room can be highly distracting to them. The sound of the air conditioner or cars on the street outside the building may make it difficult for them to hear their immediate conversation. When an autistic person does not respond to commands, do not assume they cannot hear. The background noise may be too much for them. On the other hand, some may crave noises such as a fan, or may be calmed by environmental noise or certain music. Some people use noise reducing headphones as an environmental modification. It is common for people with ASD to have an aversion to high pitched noises, such as whistles, sirens, loud voices, or babies crying. Conversely, some are drawn to those sounds. An example is a small child who broke away from her parents and ran toward the firetruck in a parade, arms outstretched, drawn to this particular sensory input. Some considerations might include moving a person away from active noises or allowing them to have an item that creates a certain noise. Additionally, allowing for noise reducing or cancelling headphones to be worn.

Sensory distortions of the gustatory system may be dangerous. People have been known to eat substances such as dirt or consume gasoline. A teacher was heard to comment that "Teaching is the only profession where we find ourselves saying 'We don't lick the pencil sharpener'." When working with children, be certain to adjust the environment to keep unsafe and/or hazardous items out of their reach. It requires careful watch as they might be prone to chew on the tires of toy cars, or other objects. A child may attempt to drink a bottle of paint or window cleaner if it is in their line of vision. As with the enjoyment of licking or eating distasteful objects, they may be drawn to noxious smells. Some of those smells, such as car exhaust or the fumes of the truck or bus, may be dangerous and toxic to the child. Some helpful considerations would be allowing for certain foods or drinks to be consumed when needed and removing distracting smells or allowing for an item that provides a regulating odor.

Problematic sensory processing can result in tactile confusions. Individuals may feel things too strongly or not at all. This applies to the clothing they wear, the touch of another person, the room temperature, or even an extremely gentle air flow. They may feel compelled to touch another person's hair or skin or constantly be touching things around them. A touch, such as a handshake may be uncomfortable; it can feel overly painful. Barboa and Luck (2017b) discussed a young girl who had frequent meltdowns at school. The teachers noticed that meltdowns often happened on warm afternoons when the room temperature increased. To accommodate the uncomfortable environment, they experimented by allowing the young girl and all the children to open the windows and breathe cool air when they felt overheated. This easy accommodation reversed the propensity toward the meltdowns and made life more enjoyable for all involved. Tactile confusions can be dangerous when pain is involved. The person may not realize they have been seriously hurt as they may not process the pain. Conversely, they may feel a highly exaggerated level of pain resulting from a small touch. Keep in mind that tactile confusion may be compounded by the person's lack of communication skills. Considerations include allowing the person to adjust their clothing (jackets on or off), making modifications to room temperature, and allowing for personal heat or cooling devices.

The vestibular system plays a part in allowing a person to be aware of where their body is in relation to the earth. Problems in vestibular processing result in poor balance and coordination. They may have difficulty on an escalator, due to the movement. Some children may continually fall out of their chairs, or run their hand along the wall as they walk. The person may fear stairs and struggle with any platform that requires balance or rotations of their body. Being autism friendly means being aware of these struggles and offering alternatives or assistance as needed. Some considerations include being tolerant of taking stairs, an escalator, or an elevator, allowing the person's office to be on the first floor, and being tolerant of certain devices such as a special chair that helps regulate vestibular input.

Understanding of the proprioceptive system shows why some children play very roughly or appear to be quite awkward. This should not be mistaken for bad behavior. Those who struggle in this sensory area often bump into others without realizing why it happened. It is difficult for them to know where their body is in relation to the space around them and one body part to another. It is important to be sensitive to the fact that the person may have bruises which are often the result of falling, clumsiness, or self-injurious behaviors. Barboa and Luck (2017a) described it as trying to navigate a crowd with a large bag hanging from the shoulder. It would be common to bump into people and things until getting used to carrying the bag. After a time, the brain adjusts to the space needed to navigate and the person stops bumping into things. Those who struggle with proprioceptive issues cannot naturally "adjust" to the knowledge of their body in relation to the space around and often require intervention and understanding. Considerations might include extra space to move and navigate, allowing a certain type of sitting arrangement such as an exercise ball, and being tolerant of unexpected bumps into other people.

Although many people have never heard of interoception, it has a large effect on the behaviors of people with autism. Interoception is the sense of what is happening inside one's own body. The body sends messages to the brain concerning hunger, thirst, sleep, bathroom needs, pain, itch, body temperature, nausea, and other bodily signals. Interoception also allows us to feel various emotions. Autistic people may not receive those signals in the same way as neurotypical individuals. This can create a situation where potty-training may be extremely delayed because the body is not signaling the needs to the brain, a person may over- or under-eat, and an individual may not notice an internal pain or injury. Do not assume that behavior is a result of a purposeful control motive. Sleep disturbances, the inability to regulate emotions, inappropriate laughter, etc. may be out of the individual's awareness and ability to manage. Considerations would include being tolerant of a person's personal schedule – going to the bathroom, eating, etc. when they discover they need to even though it might not be at a convenient or socially scheduled time.

Autism Friendly Awareness

What may seem like a simple definition of autism friendly – "being aware of social engagement and environmental factors affecting people with ASD by modifying communication methods and physical space to better suit an individual's unique and special needs." It is actually comprehensive and requires understanding combined with individualized application of strategies. Being autism friendly requires the synthesis of education and awareness with action and application. The autism friendly professional is keenly open to a continuous journey of growth and understanding about those around them who manifest with autism.

The IBCCES (2020) stated the most important thing to understand about persons with autism is that while there is a set of similarities, each person is unique. There are some generalities that apply, such as the fact that the individuals do experience sensory stimuli in a different manner than their neurotypical peers and will likely be challenged with some level of social interaction ability. A person who has taken the time and effort to learn to be autism friendly will know what the specific struggles may be and are prepared for what to expect. An individual or members of an agency or business can learn to prevent uncomfortable situations as they learn to be autism friendly. This knowledge and preparation allow businesses and community agencies to serve the neurodiverse population. With knowledge of autism friendly principles, churches can welcome all congregants, stores and restaurants can enjoy an expanded customer base, and communities can serve all citizens. This does not occur without effort; it must be recognized that families need support, and the communities and businesses need education (Barboa and Luck, 2017a).

Virtually every community in the United States has autistic citizens. As ASD is the fastest growing developmental disorder in the world today, municipalities must learn to serve all citizens. They must be inclusive for this fast-growing population. Churches and other places of worship must understand how to welcome persons with disabilities and their families. Retail establishments and restaurants can benefit from expanding their services to be inclusive to those who are differently abled. Businesses and agencies can be successful in serving individuals and families with autism by better understanding families affected by ASD. Families that include a person with autism often have added stresses associated with that challenge. Autism Action Partnership (2020) reported that the costs to raise a child with autism range from $1.4 million to $2.5 million, including medical costs, special therapies, and schooling. This is in comparison to $233,610 to raise a neurotypical child. Autism Speaks (2020) confirmed that the cost of raising a special needs child is double that of raising a neurotypical child. Financial stressors are one of many factors that can affect a family dealing with autism.

Families affected by ASD may be dealing with many challenges and stressors. Sleep deprivation of both the child and the parents is a typical factor which can affect the entire family. Parents can often feel judged when they venture out into the community and can be the victims of insults and hurtful comments by the uninformed, especially if their child is experiencing dysregulation or non-accepted social interactions. Therefore, they often avoid outings to parks, shopping, or even to church. Siblings may be affected by the fact that parental time and resources are largely directed to the needs of the family member with autism, or siblings may take on a parentified role, becoming mini caretakers in the family.

As individuals in communities become familiar with the basics of ASD, they will learn to avoid giving unsolicited advice to the parent of an autistic child, even well-intended advice about diets, cures, behavior management, or treatments. They will learn to not ask what caused the autism or make comments about the child looking "normal." They will learn to not ask if the individual has special savant skills, like "Rain Man" in the movie or another reference from a TV show. They will not pretend to know exactly what this family is going through and will not make statements such as, "God never gives us more than we can handle." They will listen to what the family is saying about the best way to serve them and the individual with ASD. They will hear the family as they alert the listener to what calms the person or what irritates them, and what may cause a sensory overload. The simplest rule to follow in relating to families with a neurodiverse family member is to be respectful of the families and refrain from being judgmental.

Being autism friendly means understanding how an individual and a family are affected by autism. It means taking the time to know a specific family and understand their unique needs and struggles, and making an effort to support. In the words of Sandy Nicholson, author, speaker, and autism advocate,

> As you go about your life each day, you will encounter many people. Some will appear to be well-behaved, and others may not. You will cross paths with people struggling to deal with a myriad of frustrations. Communication problems and sensory issues may overwhelm them.
>
> When you walk through your world today, I hope you can remain non-judgmental when you encounter a person having a hard time. Remember, they may not be misbehaving, but may have autism and be overwhelmed.
>
> Please be understanding and refrain from making judgments. Your reaction may mean the world to the parent and the child.
>
> (Barboa & Luck, 2017a, p. 46)

The *Autism Friendly Training Program* set forth in this book is foundationally set in the autism friendly definition defined in this chapter. It was developed to meet the needs of families around the world living with autism. Millions of families who have a family member with autism struggle financially, socially, and medically. Many feel judged by others, and feel ostracized by society. Often, they give up, withdraw, and discontinue taking their families to stores, restaurants, parks, and community events. Barack Obama, the 44th President of the United States, proclaimed on World Autism Awareness Day, "The greatness of our nation lies in the diversity of our people . . . Together we can create a world free of barriers to inclusion and full of understanding and acceptance of the differences that make us strong" (White House Archives, 2015). The *Autism Friendly Training Program* provides guidance on how to become inclusive and free from social and physical barriers that block equal opportunities for all autism citizens.

Although society as a whole is beginning to be more aware of autism, there remains far too much misinformation. Misperceptions are rampant and damaging. Ableism is becoming a problem. People are searching for credible answers to "What is autism?" which has been one of the most popular searches on Google in recent years (Povey, 2014). The *Autism Friendly Training Program* meets the need to create a better way of life for those with ASD. It provides an organized, accurate training tool for the professional to feel confident and able to provide healthy interactions with autistic individuals.

The *Autism Friendly Training Program* presented in this book is a fully encompassing presentation. It ranges from general information that pertains to everyone, to very specific details to assist various groups. There is also information specific to helping children understand autism. This teaches children from preschool age through high school to understand ASD and children who present with non-neurotypical characteristics. The authors have listed resources which others have found helpful, specifically for children. The award-winning children's presentations in this program are entertaining and engaging and have received acclaim from children, parents, and teachers. The *Autism Friendly* presentations have been successful for small groups, as well as for large student assemblies. The program is designed to enable the autism friendly presenter to do a generalized presentation to a diverse group of people, or to give audiences a more specific presentation. It is easily tailored to meet the needs of law enforcement, firefighters, the medical community, teachers of all levels, school support staff, restaurant personnel, colleges and universities, beauticians, businesses, employers, civic groups, community groups, extended families, churches, and children of all ages.

The *Autism Friendly Training Program* requires a group effort. The first step is to reach out to other like-minded people in a community who are interested in improving the quality of life for those with ASD. A small group can quickly grow to a larger group, which makes the commitments more manageable. The program began with four dedicated people, and has expanded to helping people around the world. As the authors have shared their knowledge and materials with others, this generosity has been reciprocated by the exchange of information and creation of further ideas and development to a more autism friendly world.

There are multiple benefits to those who participate in the *Autism Friendly Training Program*. Learning to be autism friendly is the tip of the iceberg for the attendees. The cities that have undergone the *Autism Friendly City Program* have been amazed at the positive media promotion which resulted. Following the training, some cities have received inquiries from around the world of people interested in moving to their community. Restaurants have reported an increased income by serving families who have a member with special needs. City programs have reported positive feedback after implementing program modifications which allow autistic individuals and their families to take part in community events. Churches have been enthusiastic about extending their reach and better serving the autistic, population. Families have been enthusiastic about this program, which has been truly life- changing to many. Those who have felt very alone have discovered a chance to meet others and feel connected. Families have the opportunity to enjoy the company of people without feeling judged, or feeling the need to stay home. By employing the multi-faceted definition, the *Autism Friendly Training Program* has the potential to change lives in many ways, opening the world for families. The professionals educating themselves on this material will be leading that process, as understanding the definition presented here establishes a knowledge base and provides a roadmap to the goal of becoming autism friendly.

7 The Autism Friendly Training Program

The Presentation

The goal of the *Autism Friendly Training Program* is to offer training to all citizens to educate them about ASD. The learner objective is to identify physical and social barriers and become aware of how to better address the needs of those with autism. Awareness and understanding of ASD have improved markedly in recent times. However, there is still much progress to be made. Misperceptions and stigma about autism are rampant and damaging. Knowledge is the key to eliminating misperceptions and stigmas and the *Autism Friendly Training Program* provides a concise, organized tool to spread that knowledge.

The previous chapters in this book presented basics about autism. This chapter will allow you to take the basic understanding about ASD and present information to others in a formalized autism friendly presentation. The information given about challenges in sensory, communication, and social skills is formatted here into a concise training presentation that may be utilized to teach various groups of learners to become autism friendly. While it is important to enlighten the population about autism, the availability of competent and knowledgeable presenters is scant. This chapter provides an overview of the main components to be covered in an *Autism Friendly Training*. This information serves as a practical tool for presenters wanting to teach others or individuals wanting to increase their own knowledge.

Using the following format, the autism friendly presenter will verbally provide important facts along with points of interest, short vignettes, key concepts, and general added information. To facilitate the role of the presenter facing a variety of audiences, each topic introduced may include:

- *Material to be Presented* – An overview of the information that will be covered in each section of the presentation.
- *Key Points* – The most important constructs for the attendees to know are presented as key points. The presenter will want to pay special attention to addressing each of these points.
- *Talking Points* – Important and interesting concepts. These assist the learner in remembering the facts presented, and are helpful in keeping the audience engaged.

DOI: 10.4324/9781003105633-8

- *Information Specific to Emergency Responders* – These points guide the first responder to make connections to the general material.
- *Information Specific to Educators* – These points guide the educator to make connections to the general material. These are appropriate for teachers, administrators, or other school staff.
- *Examples and Vignettes* – Suggestions will be provided to further clarify the points as they are presented. These will help highlight the unique experience of those with ASD. As Figure 7.1 illustrates, those with autism have their own view of the world.

Presentation Topic - What is Autism?

Material to be Presented:

Autism is a complex disorder. Our brains continually collect information about the world through our senses (including vision, hearing, smell, touch, taste, proprioception, vestibular, and interoception). In autism, the senses may be over- or under-processing incoming stimuli. Autistic people are often not able to regulate sensory information. Autism can affect one or all the eight sensory areas influencing the ability to communicate, social abilities, and behavior. Most often there are impairments in executive functioning. Executive functioning skills are the abilities that allow an individual to accomplish daily tasks. Executive functions enable people to plan, organize, and complete activities. It impacts decision making, processing, attention,

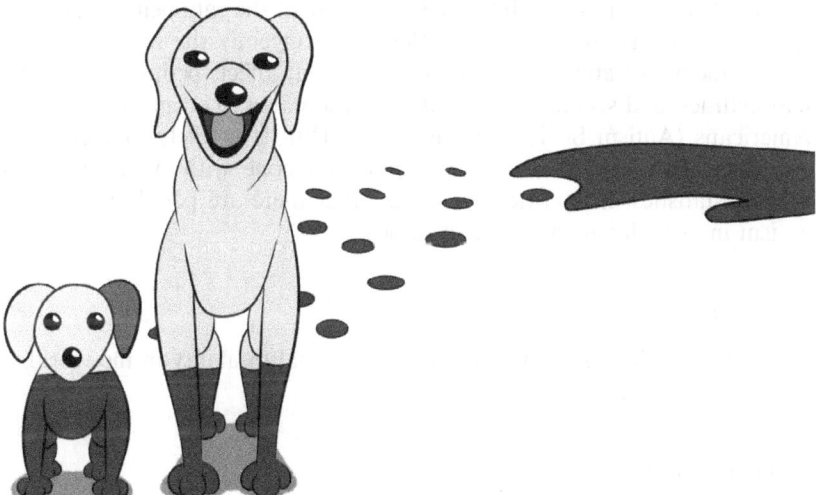

Figure 7.1 People with autism see the world from a different perspective.
Source: Illustration courtesy of Landon Kemp

time management, organizational skills, and problem solving. An extended glossary of terms referring to autism can be found in Appendix 1.

Key Points:

- ASD presents in a variety of ways; no two people are affected the same.
- The person with autism may learn easily, or conversely, still be an "early learner."
- Autism affects the ability to communicate, to process sensory information, to navigate socially, and produce acceptable behavior.
- ASD affects the ability to successfully complete activities of daily living by interfering with the ability to plan, organize, and complete tasks.

Talking Points:

- Autism is complex to understand because each person is so unique. However, there are many characteristics that are common for this population, and this presentation will focus on those.

Presentation Topic – Why Everyone Needs to Know About Autism

Material to be Presented:

The Centers for Disease Control and Prevention (CDC) (2020) currently estimates that 1 in 54 children have autism with the rate being four times more common in males than females. It is currently the fastest growing developmental disability in the United States. It affects people of all races, nationalities, and social classes. Autism is estimated to occur in 3.5 million Americans (Autism Society of America, 2020). It is likely that everyone will have association at some time with someone with ASD. With the current statistics, it is critical to realize that there are people living with autism in virtually every city in America.

Key Points:

- Autism is the fastest growing developmental disability in the world.
- 3.5 million Americans have autism.

Talking Points:

- No one knows the reason for the increase in autism diagnosis. Through this training, the mission is to help families currently affected by autism and improve quality of life for those with ASD.

Educator Points:

- A few decades ago, education majors in college were told they would likely never see an autistic child , because it was so rare. This is no longer accurate; autistic children can be found in every education setting.
- An educator's role is two-fold: to teach the child who has ASD and to teach others about autism.

Emergency Responder Points:

- It has been stated that people with autism are seven times more likely than their neurotypical peers to require the services of an emergency responder at some point in their lives. (Stelter, 2018).
- First responders can assume that an individual with autism will be their patient at some point. The more the first responder understands and is prepared for interacting with an autistic person, the more success will be achieved in the interaction.
- In many places around the country, the 911 system is the front line in meeting the needs in case of an emergency. Dispatchers are highly trained to record important data and to dispense that data to those responding. A person dialing 911 from locations where that service is available will be connected to emergency dispatchers. Some 911 service areas offer a voluntary Special Needs Assessment Form to identify homes of persons with a variety of special needs, including ASD. In those areas, if a call is made to the 911 dispatcher, information is automatically relayed about the special needs if the patron has signed the form in advance. This allows the responders to know what barriers they may face. Caregivers of individuals with autism may have installed extra locks or bars on doors if elopement is an issue. The first responder may be coming into a situation where a child may bolt, or where there could be communication difficulties. The responder may be alerted if the resident is prone to bolting or does not respond to verbal directives. If the patient or another person in the home is autistic, the first responder will have a more successful entry if they can get this information in advance. The responders might decide to avoid use of their emergency sirens and lights, which could cause escalation of an incident if a person with autism is involved. As Figure 7.2 illustrates, communication and sensory challenges can be problematic. A quieter, less visual approach might avoid escalating the situation. For a sample Special Needs Assessment Form, see Appendix 3.

Presentation Topic – What are the Main Challenges Associated with Autism?

Material to be Presented:

An autistic individual can face many challenges and their autism can manifest in many ways. The core features of autism include communication

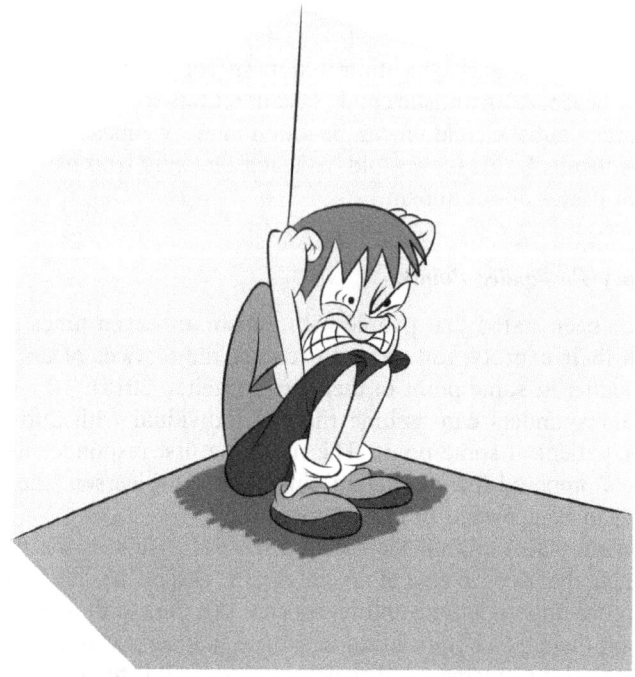

Figure 7.2 Communication and sensory struggles equal behaviors
Source: Illustration courtesy of Landon Kemp

(verbal and nonverbal) struggles, sensory processing issues, difficulty in social interactions, and what may seem to others as a presentation of odd or unusual behaviors. There can certainly be additional considerations and the professional will need to remember that each person with ASD will present with their own struggle areas and nuances.

Talking Points:

- A person's communication and sensory challenges can result in problematic behaviors. The struggles and the behavior reactions may not make sense to the neurotypical observer (Obrey, 2019).

Presentation Topic – How are Communication Skills Affected?

Material to be Presented:

Communication is our most basic connection to others in our world. When the ability to communicate effectively is missing, this interferes with a full and happy life. Although some people with autism may have advanced language skills, others may be severely language delayed. It is important to remember that just because a person is nonverbal does not mean they cannot understand what is being said. It is common for autistic individuals to have uneven skills in receptive (taking in) language and expressive (putting out) language. One area may be high while the other area is exceptionally low. Communication skills can be affected in many ways.

Key Points:

- Individuals with ASD may lack a social "filter" – they may say what they think although the comment may be inappropriate or hurtful.

  a. A child may state that someone is fat, ugly, or has a bald spot. The autistic child may tell another child that a picture the other child drew is ugly or they may verbally express they do not like it. This is not to be cruel, but they tend to tell the truth as they see it, with little regard for feelings of others or social norms.

- They may be delayed in language development.

  a. As an adult or teenager, they may have the language skills of a noticeably younger child.
  b. They may remain basically nonverbal or use words or sounds that have no functional meaning. Or, they may have advanced language and sound like a little professor when they speak.

- They may repeat words, phrases, or entire paragraphs they have heard before.

  a. Jayden repeated the words, "Two weeks!" on a regular basis for years.
  b. Another child could repeat the entire script from Lion King movie at age three and this was their primary way of speaking to others.
  c. Little Alexis would imitate people's laughter or mimic the cry of a baby when she heard it.
  d. When Timmy would enter class, he would repeat phrases from old TV shows. A fan of Gilligan's Island, he would greet the teacher each day with "Ahoy, Matey!"
  e. A man with autism was a student at a day-service center. A volunteer was trying to assemble a swing set and the adult student was allowed to help. The volunteer did not know that the student had autism manifesting with language/communication issues. The student would point to sections of the laid-out equipment and say, "That's the top" repeatedly, causing the volunteer to rearrange the pieces that were laid out on the ground. Soon the volunteer grew weary and complained to the staff of the center, "This student isn't much help!" The staff

realized they had not told the volunteer that the only two things the student would say all day were, "That's the top" and, "chicken."

- They may speak in a flat tone of voice with little to no inflection.
- They may have difficulty constructing sentences.

  a. A mom tells a story that they took their family to a local amusement park where a height requirement is listed for each ride. When their pre-teen aged nonverbal son attempted to board a ride, the attendant informed them that the boy was too short for this ride. The son, who as yet had never spoken, loudly proclaimed his displeasure by saying, "Well, that is BULL****!" Others looked on, shocked by the language, as this family celebrated the son's accomplishment of communication.

- They may use some basic sign language or an electronic communication device.
- They may have difficulty understanding what is said to them.

  a. There can be difficulty with words or phrases that have two meanings. When Patti's boys were being boisterous with a toy car at the dinner table, she told them to, "Knock it off!" So, they did, hitting the car right onto the floor.

- They may have difficulty expressing themselves clearly, understanding what others say to them, or require extra time to process what others are saying.
- They may have difficulty understanding all-inclusive words, such as everyone, no one, always, never, all, and none.

  a. When Katrina was small, the gym teacher was frustrated that Katrina refused to follow directions, such as, "Everybody run!" After the teacher understood that Katrina does not identify as "everybody," the teacher began saying "Everybody and Katrina, run!" The problem was solved.

Talking Points:

- Individuals may have problems communicating verbally and non-verbally.
- As illustrated in Figure 7.3, they may use alternate methods to communicate.
- They might understand more than they can express, or express language at a higher level than they can understand.
- Autistic individuals often take what is said literally, and view language in more concrete terms.
- They may repeat words, phrases, or paragraphs.

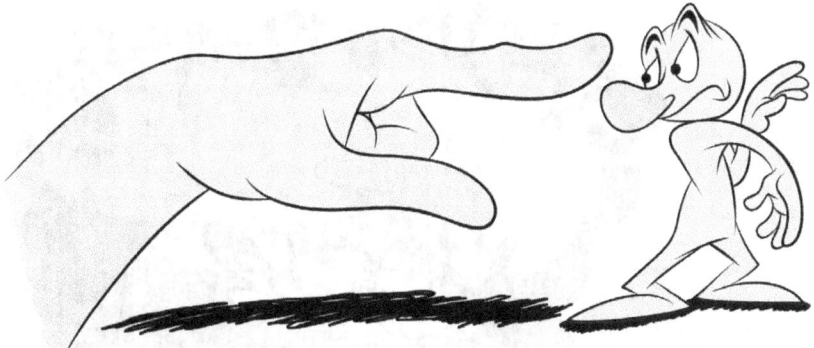

Figure 7.3 People with autism may use communication methods other than speech.
Source: Illustration courtesy of Landon Kemp

- They often do not understand "all-inclusive" words or generic words.
- Autistic individuals usually understand more than they can express but can also talk at a level that does not match their understanding.
- They may use communication methods other than speech (sign language or an electronic device).
- When speaking to someone with ASD, say what is meant. Avoid idioms and figures of speech as illustrated in Figure 7.4.

    a. Example: When asked to bring in the leaves to extend the table for a large dinner gathering, the children brought in leaves from a tree.
    b. When given instructions to bake brownies using "two whole eggs," a teenage girl included the egg shells.

- A class of children did a particularly great job one day and the teacher complimented them by saying, "You're on fire today!" They were frightened, ran, and screamed.
- When Willow was little, her mother had a well-established bedtime routine for her. However, when Willow's daddy would attempt the bedtime routine, things would explode and end in chaos. One night, the mom listened from around the corner and it seemed that Daddy followed the routine quite well. After bath, a drink of water, and a story, he told Willow "OK, now jump in bed." She did exactly as she was told, and gleefully began jumping on the bed.
- Word confusion may stem from words with double meanings, from idioms, or from misunderstanding a word or phrase. A mother reported that her son refused to say the Pledge of Allegiance at school. He was a bright boy, and no one could figure out why he became so upset each morning during the pledge, causing chaos in the classroom. He explained it this way, "I know what a widget is, but I don't know what

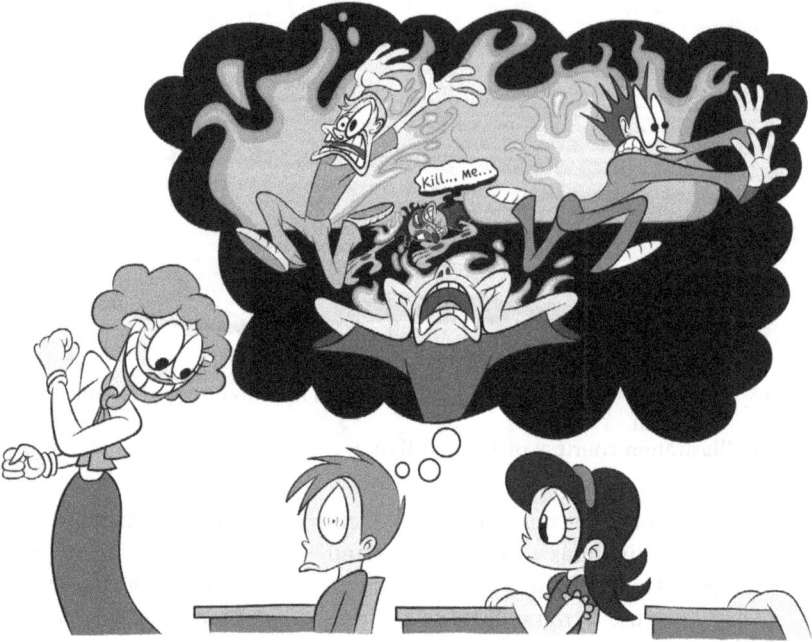

Figure 7.4 People with autism may not understand figures of speech
Source: Illustration courtesy of Landon Kemp

a widget stand is. I don't want to pledge my allegiance to the 'Republic for Widget Stands.'"

- Avoid teasing and joking, as those with ASD often process things literally and may struggle with humor.
- If the person seems to not understand what is said, change the wording. Do not simply repeat the exact same words, and do not speak louder. People with autism often have a variety of communication issues which make it difficult to not only speak, but also to understand what is being said to them.
- Keep directions simple. Giving multi-step directions may be confusing.
- The person may not understand facial expressions or body language and it is often helpful to include pointing and gesturing.

Educator Points:

- Be clear, state directions in the positive rather than the negative, and avoid long verbiage and/or dialogue.

    a. Rather than saying, "Don't run," say, "Walk." They may have a short attention span and only remember the last word. They may hear that they are being told not to run, but not know what to do instead, so they may begin jumping or skipping. Tell them what they need to do.

b. Do not take it personally if the child does not seem to use "friendly" communication. They are challenged trying to survive in a world that makes little sense to them.

c. Autistic children may have difficulty with pronouns and prepositions. A special needs preschool class was having show-and-tell with each child's favorite toy. At the end of the activity, the teacher said, "Now, run and put the toys up." They all began running around the class while holding the toys in the air.

d. Give direct instruction rather than indirect instruction. Rather than saying, "Your face is dirty," say, "Wash your face." Instead of saying, "We can't go outside until all the centers are cleaned up" say, "Put the blocks away." It is difficult for the individual to infer your wishes when they hear an indirect statement.

e. Give directives in the form of a statement, not a question. Rather than saying, "Are you ready to come to circle time now?" say, "Come to circle time now." They may not understand that the question being asked is actually a directive, and they may simply answer the question rather than comply with the request.

f. A music teacher was exasperated with a boy who was having an outburst. The boy was shouting, "The teacher is a liar! She says I NEVER stay in my chair and says I am ALWAYS talking. That's not true! Sometimes I do stay in my chair, and sometimes I am not talking." When the teacher understood the communication barrier, they and the student were better able to work together.

Emergency Responder Points:

• Sensory processing is often challenged in autisitc people. This includes neurologically processing what is being heard. When speaking to them, it may take them more time than expected to process and understand what is being said. Give them time to think about what was said and to provide a response. When the questions or directives are given in rapid succession, they may become increasingly confused and not be able to respond. Be patient, pause, and wait for a slower processing speed.

• Provide direct instructions to those with ASD. They often will not understand indirect instruction.

a. For example, do not say, "I need to look in your mouth now." Rather, say, "Open your mouth." Instead of saying, "I can't wrap this bandage on your leg while you are kicking," say, "Hold your leg still."

    b.   When told, "Go into the other room and sit down," they may sit right down where they are because they may only attend to the last thing they hear.

- Explain the use of the flashlight, tongue depressor, and other medical tools, perhaps letting the individual touch the tools before they are used.
- If there is a behavioral issue involved, autism friendly communication is the first strategy to de-escalate the situation.
- Communicating with the caregiver will provide vital information about the person's abilities and how their reactions and communication abilities may be different from a neurotypical person.
- Be alert to the use of all-inclusive or generic words in any directives.

    a.   Rather than saying "Everyone stand over here," if suspecting the person has autism, tell them directly, "Jimmy, stand by the door."

    b.   If you refer to the person in generic terms, such as "Son" or "Buddy," they may not know the reference is to them.

- Learn the basic signs for words such as "pain," and "where?" This can serve as a valuable tool in communication. Basic sign language can be learned for free on the internet from YouTube channels such as Bill Vicars (2017).

Presentation Topic – Understanding Families Affected by ASD

Material to be Presented:

The stress of autism can impact the entire family. Often families are stressed with the challenges that ASD can present in both the home and school settings. Families of children with autism regularly report being sleep deprived, as children may suffer from sleep disorders and parents struggle to find time for adequate amounts of sleep. Taking an autistic child into the community can be difficult and stressful for the family. Others often stare, criticize, fail to understand behaviors that occur, and make hurtful comments to the family. The time and resources that a family directs toward the child with autism may take away from siblings and create an imbalance in parental attention. This can lead to resentment issues with neurotypical siblings.

Key Points:

- Families affected by autism have a high degree of stress due to financial, medical, educational, and social concerns.
- Many of these families may be experiencing sleep deprivation and little to no self-care.

- Families may avoid outings that most families enjoy such as a trip to the park, shopping, going to a restaurant, a school event, or attending church.

Talking Points:

- Understanding the issues families face when parenting a child with ASD can help the professional provide better empathy and service.
- Grant (2017a) highlighted many of the ways families can be affected by autism, including financial stressors from treatments and therapies, social isolation, lack of respite care, extended family members not understanding ASD, waiting lists for treatments, worrying about the future after the parents are gone, education struggles and being kicked out of school, a 24/7 parenting attention/hypervigilance on prevention, a highly scheduled and consistent routine with little flexibility, and marriage stressors.

Emergency Responder Points:

- Autistic children often have other medical complications adding to the stress experienced by families. Some parents may be dealing with a trauma response from parenting a child with ASD. Some autistic children have a parent with autism who is struggling with their own issues.

Presentation Topic – Communicating with Caregivers

Material to be Presented:

Parents and caregivers of children with autism understand their child the best, yet often receive a great deal of unsolicited advice about how to raise their child. Professionals should listen to what the caregiver says about the child with autism. The family is the 24/7 team and knows the child better than anyone else does. Parents can explain what calms the child, what agitates them, and typically how to best handle the child in problematic situations. When communicating with parents and caregivers do not give unsolicited advice about discipline, diets, treatments, or "cures" and do not comment on the child looking "normal." Speak as you would with any other child, such as, "Your hair looks pretty today" or, "I like that blue shirt." Also avoid asking if the child is a genius, a savant, or has special skills. Do not ask parents what caused the autism and do not claim to know exactly what the parent is going through. Effective communication also involves avoiding comments such as "God never gives us more than we can handle" or "You must be such a special person for God to give you a special child."

Key Points:

- Be respectful of all families. Refrain from being judgmental and try to listen and gain understanding.
- Communicate with the awareness that the parent is the expert on their child.
- Avoid giving your own opinions, thoughts, and suggestions unless solicited from the parent.

Educator Points:

- If a parent describes a problem they are having with the child, do not say, "They do not do that at school." Rather than being comforting to the parent, many will find this demeaning and accusatory.
- Ask the parent what is rewarding to the child and what disturbs them. Gain awareness about the child through the parent's expertise.
- Communicate with a goal to become a partner with the parents.

Emergency Responder Points:

- If searching for a lost child, ask the caregivers what the child is drawn to and what they avoid.
- A child with autism may be drawn to water. This is a typical manifestation and unfortunately many lost autistic children have been found drowned in a pond or river.
   a. A 911 manager reported a call came in about a lost child with autism. The 911 manager had learned that these children may be drawn to water. The dispatcher sent a team to the home but sent a second team to the nearby creek where they found the child by the water's edge.
- The child may be hiding to avoid loud noises, crowds, or some other sensory overload. As illustrated in Figure 7.5, this is a significant issue with autism.
- Many children with ASD will become dysregulated being around new or unfamiliar people or new surroundings such as an ambulance or police car.

Presentation Topic – What do the Senses Have to do with Autism?

Material to be Presented:

Distorted sensory perception is a common component of autism. The way a person with ASD perceives the world around them is different from the way neurotypical individuals take in information from the environment.

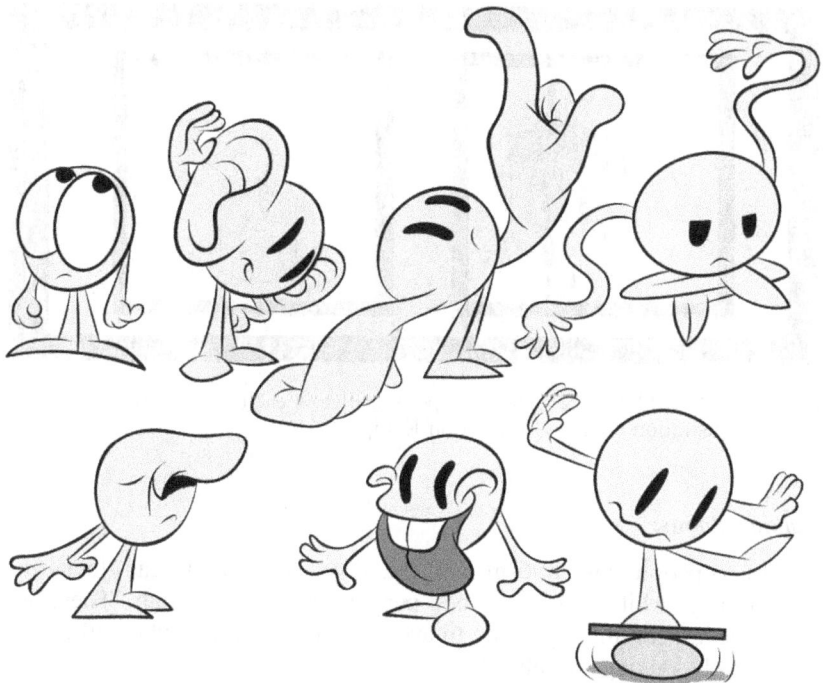

Figure 7.5 Distorted sensory perception is a major part of autism
Source: Illustration courtesy of Landon Kemp

An autistic person's sense of taste can differ from the preferences of friends
or family members and the difference can be highly exaggerated. Hearing,
touch, smell, and vision sensitivities vary among the general population
and those with autism can represent the far reaches to each end of that
distribution. What would be generally experienced by others without discomfort in sound, visual, etc. levels in the environment can be felt in the
extreme by those with autism. Sight, hearing, taste, smell, and touch may
all mesh together with sensitivities in multiple areas.

Key Points:

- One or more of the senses may be affected.
- Sensory challenges can vary from day to day, even minute to minute.
- Behavior manifestations may be the individual's effort to avoid a certain sensation or to seek more sensory input from the world around
  them. Figure 7.6 illustrates how a person can be hypo- or
  hypersensitive.
- The autistic person may get erroneous signals from their own receptors about what is happening in their own body.

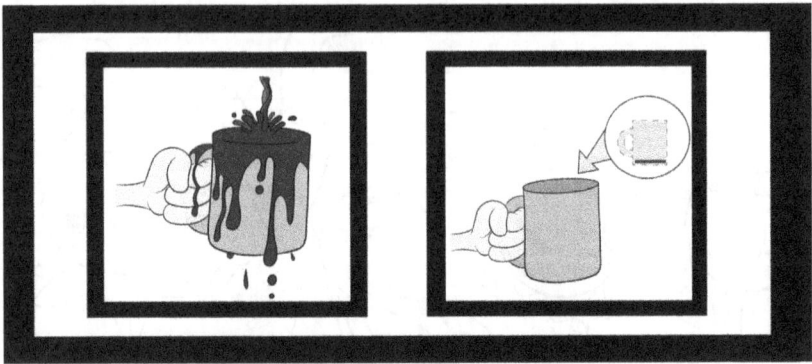

Figure 7.6 A child may be hypo or hyper-sensitive in each sensory area
Source: Illustration courtesy of Landon Kemp

Talking Points:

- Some people with autism feel, see, taste, smell, and hear things too strongly, while others do not perceive strongly enough. Therefore, some are continually trying to avoid incoming stimuli while others are actively seeking stimuli.

  a. Think of it like 2 cups. Some people have a very large sensory cup and they work continually to fill that cup. They cannot seem to get enough of a certain sense. Others have a very small sensory cup and it is quickly filled and overloaded.

- One or more of the senses may be affected. It is not uncommon for someone with sensory challenges to have difficulties in multiple areas. The level the individual perceives of each type of stimuli in their environment may change continually.

- Vision Sensory Area: Struggles in sensory processing of visual stimuli may result in the person either being too sensitive to light and other visual stimuli and needing to wear sunglasses indoors as illustrated in Figure 7.7, or not sensitive enough. Eye contact may be disturbing to the individual. They may be confused or get upset by rapid movements in their line of vision, or random movements.

  a. Professionals attempting to engage a person with ASD may find it helpful to physically approach gently and explain any movements before they are made.

  b. Movement such as people walking or shopping carts being pushed can be very upsetting, as the movements blurs together.

  c. They may rely on visual cues other than facial recognition. When a well-known teacher walked past the school room window, the little boy inside the school asked, "Where is that green shirt going?"

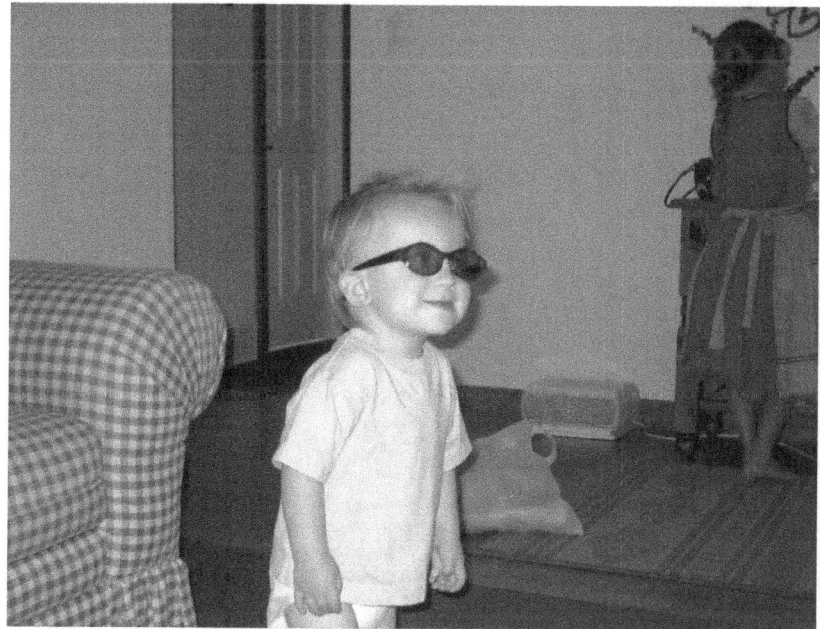

Figure 7.7 The sense of vision may be affected in various ways
Source: Photo courtesy of E. Obrey

    d. Another child walked down the hall at school. When they passed the speech room, they looked up in surprise and said, "Oh, hi, Mrs. Wyatt, I didn't know it was you until I saw your blue shoes."

    e. Many children feel strong visual pleasure in reaction to certain colors. If Aiden misbehaves, his parents slowly start removing all blue items from the line of sight in the living room. He will behave when the replacement of the blue items is his reward.

- Hearing Sensory Area: Struggles in hearing sensory processing can result in the person being either too sensitive to sound in the environment or not sensitive enough. Professionals may find it helpful to move to a quiet area to reduce the person's agitation. When treating a person who seems to not respond to voice, do not increase to a shouting level. Continue to use a calm voice, possibly using different words. When a person does not respond to commands, do not assume they cannot hear. One disturbing aspect may be background noise that is perceived to be as prominent as the voice of the person they are trying to listen to. Noises emanating from outside the conversation such as the sound of a heater, lights, or fans, can all be disturbing.

    a. An example is a doorbell. The person may not even seem to hear it one day, and another day may cover their ears, as illustrated in Figure 7.8, and scream in pain when they hear it.

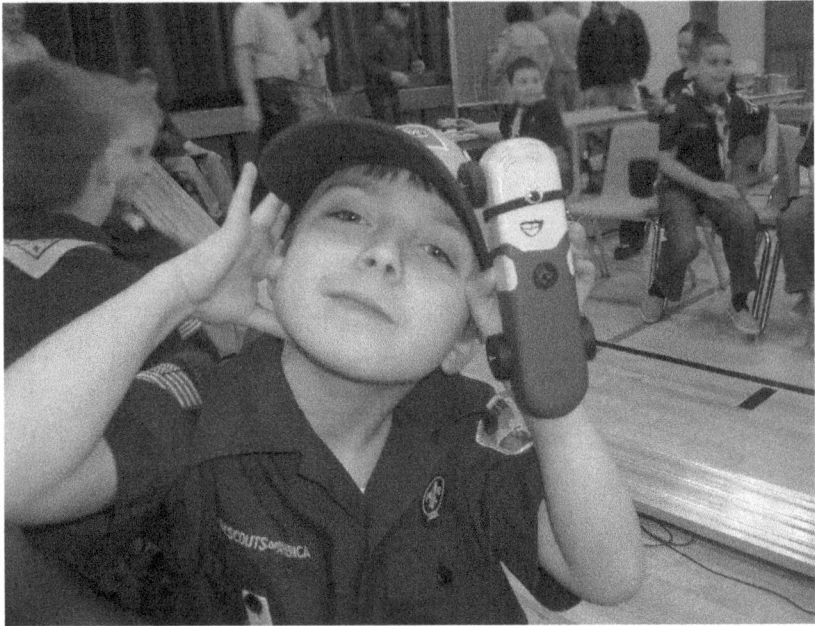

Figure 7.8 Auditory sensitivities may be experienced
Source: Photo courtesy of E. Obrey

    b.   When Emma was a toddler, she broke from her mother's hand while watching a parade. As the local fire truck came along, siren blasting, she ran to the fire truck with outstretched arms, hoping to hug the truck.

    c.   When Oliver was young, he would stick crayons in his ears to serve as earplugs to muffle classroom noise.

    d.   Those with auditory sensory struggles may wear noise reducing headphones to neutralize sounds.

- Taste Sensory Area: Struggles in taste sensory processing may distort a person's perception of things they taste. Items may seem tasteless or far too intense. A distorted sense of taste sometimes results in a person ingesting a harmful substance, such as poisonous mixtures.

    a.   Think about how one person's taste preferences differ from that of their friends and family. People with autism may have very strong sensitivities to taste and this affects their preferences as illustrated in Figure 7.9.

    b.   Often autistic persons have an extremely limited variety of foods they will eat. Many parents say their children will only eat about four different foods.

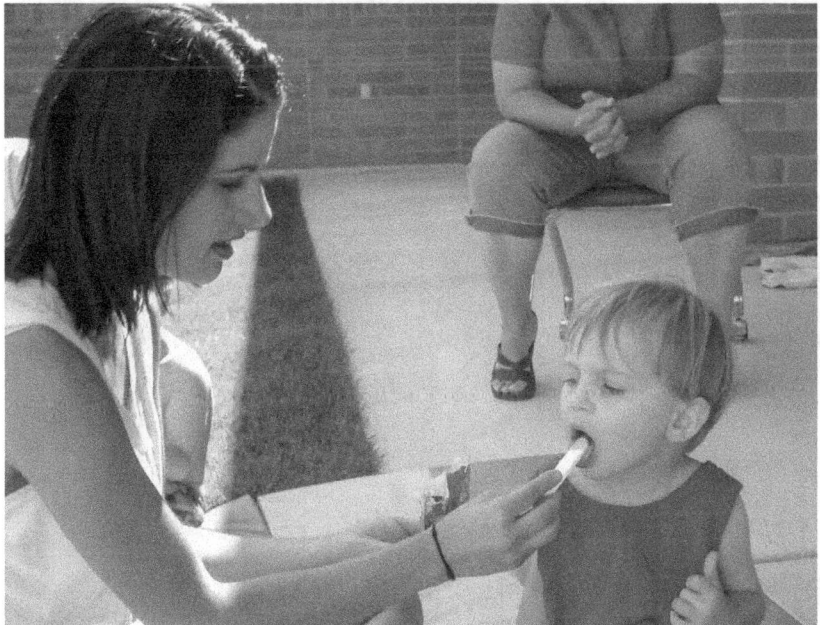

Figure 7.9 Items may seem to be tasteless or too intense in taste
Source: Photo courtesy of E. Obrey

    c. When Sophia was very young, her parents gave her a piece of citrus-flavored candy. Sophia said, "It tastes like sunshine."

    d. A person with autism may have pica, a disorder characterized by a compulsion to eat non-edible objects, such as dirt and paper.

- Smell Sensory Area: Struggles in smell sensory processing may result in odors being far too intense or the absence of noticing an odor. They may be repulsed by the smell of items that normally are not noticed by others, or they may be drawn to noxious odors.

    a. Those with sensory struggles may want to sniff another person's skin or hair or other object as illustrated in Figure 7.10.

    b. As a flight was boarding a plane, a family of four stood in the line. The little girl was complaining to her mother, "Mom! Jax is smelling my hair again!"

    c. A teacher told about a boy who kept backing up when she would talk to him. He explained he hated the smell of her breath after she had been drinking coffee. He stated he liked her breath when it smelled like peppermint.

    d. Mateo hates the smell of flowers. It is repulsive to him but seems to like the smell of chemicals.

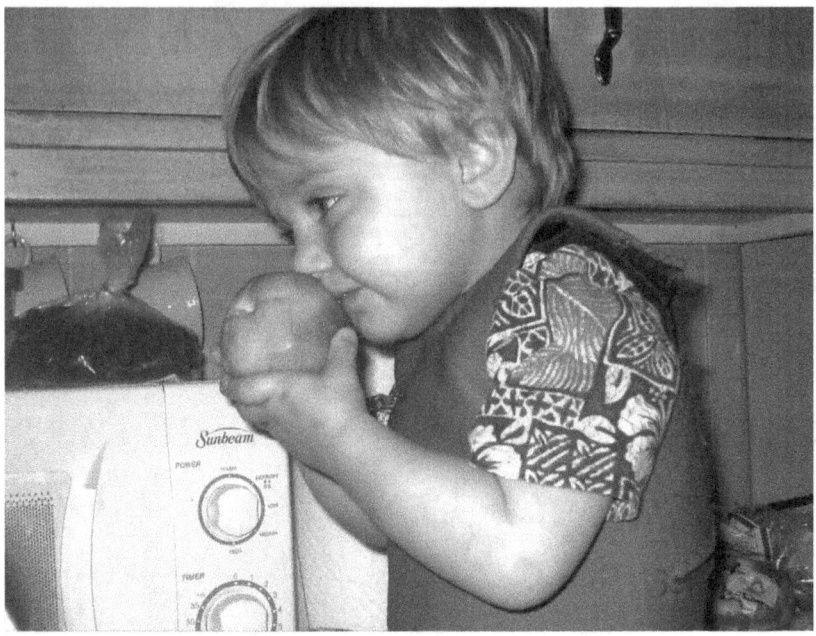

Figure 7.10 The sense of smell may be distorted

- Feeling and Touch Sensory Area: As illustrated in Figure 7.11, struggles in touch sensory processing can result in not feeling things enough or feeling them too strongly. This may apply to grabbing something, clothing, someone touching the person, or even the sensation of air.

  a. Often a light touch is more disturbing to them than a firm touch, but a person can have sensitivities either way.

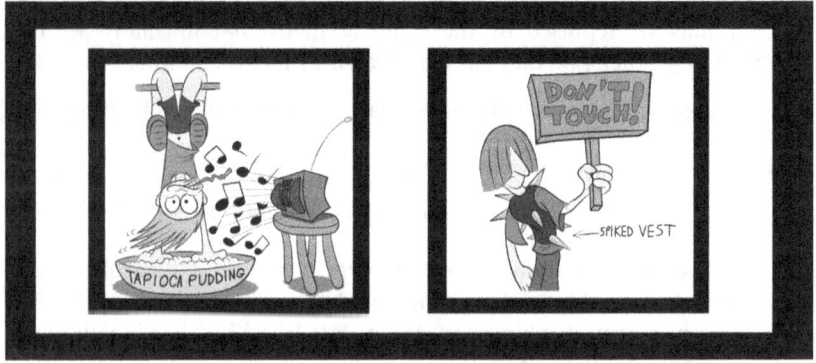

Figure 7.11 A person with ASD may avoid or seek tactile stimulation
Source: Illustration courtesy of Landon Kemp

    b. Think about the act of shaking hands with another person; that touch may be perceived as too firm or too slight. This could also be the case with a high five or a pat on the back.

- Along with the five senses that have been discussed, there are three additional senses that may be affected in autistic people – vestibular, proprioceptive, and interoceptive.
- Vestibular Sensory Area: Struggles in vestibular sensory processing affect the sense of knowing where the body is in relation to the earth (see Figure 7.12). Poor vestibular processing results in poor balance

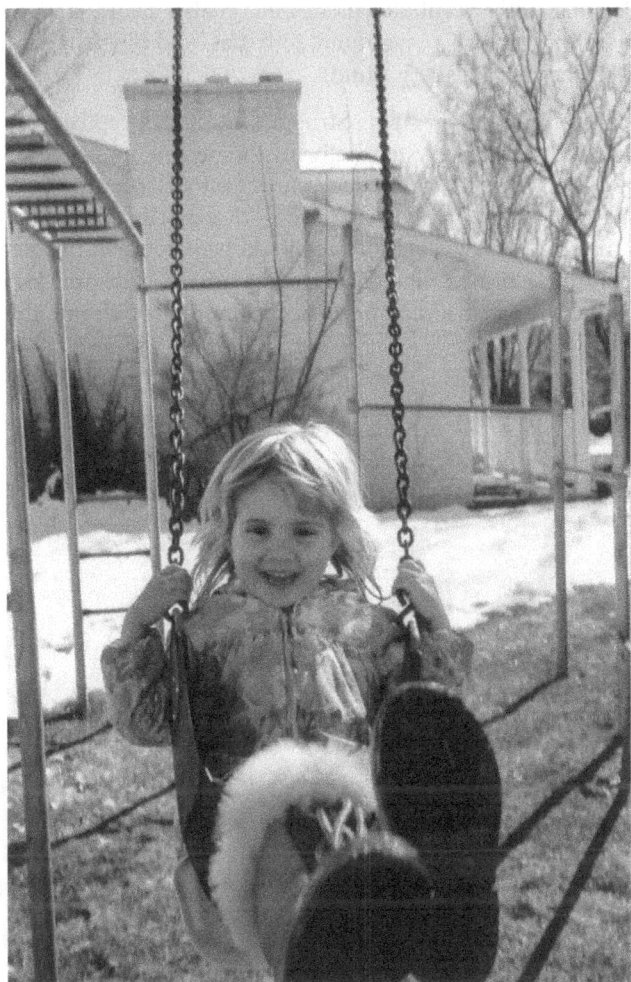

Figure 7.12 The vestibular sense is knowing where the body is in relation to the earth
Source: Photo courtesy of E. Obrey

and coordination. People with autism may have a severe reaction of claustrophobia if they are put into a small space, or if there are a lot of people crowding around.

   a.   An EMS provider who completed the autism friendly training told of responding to a call concerning a child with autism. As the medical team began to gather, the child was heading into a meltdown due to the crowd gathering. The EMT suggested they all wait in the adjoining room, with only one EMT and the mom having hands on the patient. The child immediately calmed and responded to treatment.

   b.   Persons with vestibular issues may also avoid and resist fast moving activities, playground activities, and physical games where their feet are off the ground.

- Proprioception Sensory Area: Struggles in proprioceptive sensory processing affect how the system informs the person about the position of their body in relation to the space around them (see Figure 7.13) and their other body parts. Poor proprioceptive processing results in clumsiness and lack of coordination. It should be noted that this person may regularly have bruises due to bumping into objects and falling. The large number of bruises must be differentiated from abuse by a caregiver.

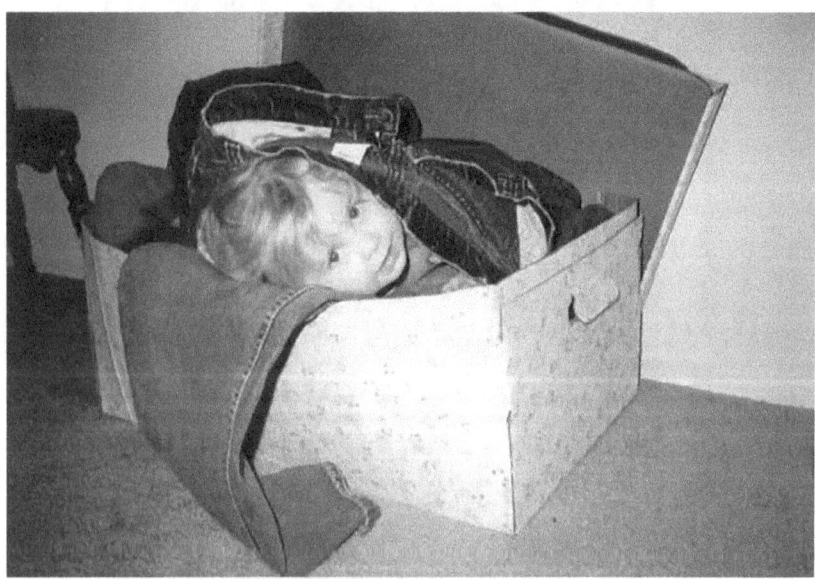

Figure 7.13 The proprioceptive sense is knowing where the body is in relation to the space around you

Source: Photo courtesy of E. Obrey

a. A person with proprioceptive difficulties may bump their head as they get into a car or regularly trip, fall, and bump into objects.

b. People with proprioceptive issues may play too roughly or appear to be clumsy. They may run into other people or hit other people unintentionally.

- Interoception Sensory Area: Struggles in interoception sensory processing affect how a person notices what is happening in their own body. Throughout each person's body are many receptors. The body sends information to the brain which allows a person to make sense of these messages, such as hunger, the need to go to the bathroom, itch, pain, body temperature, nausea, and other bodily signals. Interoception also allows individuals to feel emotions. People with autism do not receive these signals in the typical way and may have confusions about the signals their body sends the brain.

a. They may laugh inappropriately or show sleep or eating disturbances. The purpose of interoception is to drive our behavior. When a person feels hungry, they know to eat. When a person feels tired, they sleep. With interoception struggles, the person will not feel these signals.

b. A child may be slow to potty-train because they may not feel the body sensations telling them they need to "go" until it is already happening. They may also perceive urination or bowel movement as painful, causing them to resist going.

c. The feeling of hunger or thirst may be pleasant for them, causing them to not eat or drink because they do not want the pleasant feeling to go away.

d. The same may be true of the sensation to void the bowel or bladder. They may enjoy the sensation of needing to "go," so they refuse to empty their bowel or bladder.

e. Presenters can ask the participants to close their eyes and think about the stimuli they perceive from their body. Are they breathing deeply or not? Are they hungry? How do their stomachs feel? How do their muscles feel? Are they relaxed or nervous? How can they tell? What are they tapping into? These feelings remain in the "background" of our consciousness until they are needed to alert us. For autistic people, the feelings may be muted, confused, or highly exaggerated.

f. The person with autism often has difficulty interpreting what their body is trying to tell them. They may have difficulty interpreting pain, temperature, itch, sensual touch, sensations from their organs and muscles, hunger, thirst, and breathlessness.

g. A preschooler named Hudson would describe to his mother how many bowel movements were "lined up" inside his abdomen waiting to be eliminated. He could further predict which would be easy to pass and which would be a strain.

    h.   Interoceptive sensations, especially pain, may be unreliable indicators in individuals affected by autism. This sensory system can be extremely confusing for the individual and accurately reporting on internal states may be difficult.

    i.   A common minor ailment may progress to a potentially serious illness as they may not detect the early sensations. They may not be able to tell others about a serious internal issue because they cannot feel it. Also, being submerged in water may not produce a natural appropriate response - their bodies may remain passive, and they may not naturally attempt to move to the surface.

Educator Points:

- Visual stimuli may result in the person either being too sensitive to light in the classroom, the color of paint on the wall, or other visual stimuli. The person could also be not sensitive enough to visual cues such as signs and posters.
- If their visual cup is too small, the person will cover their eyes, squint, or wear sunglasses indoors, to avoid bright lights and sunlight.

    a.   They may withdraw from participating in group movement activities and they may be scared by moving objects.

    b.   They will likely avoid direct eye contact and they may have frequent headaches, dizziness, or nausea when using sight.

- If their visual cup is too large, they may stare at bright lights, even direct sunlight, as well as at moving objects.

    a.   They may move and shake their head during writing or other fine motor activities and will probably hold items closely for inspection.

    b.   They may seem unaware of new people or items in their environment.

    c.   They will frequently lose the place on a page, and they will seek visual stimulation from patterns and items that spin (such as fans).

    d.   They may also spend their recess watching the movements of their shadows in the sunlight.

- If their auditory cup is too small, they may cry, scream, or become angry at sudden noises. They may cover their ears or ask for headphones to block out noise.

    a.   They may avoid everyday noises such as a toilet flushing or water flowing. Toilets that flush automatically may be particularly distressing and scary.

    b.   High pitched noises will likely bother them, such as whistles or sirens.

- If their auditory cup is too large, they will prefer loud music and loud noises.

   a. They will always seem to use an outside voice, talking too loudly when close by others. They will also crave common noises such as an air conditioner, a fan, or water running.
   b. Those with sound sensitivities may be calmed by noises (tone or pitch) or certain music.

Emergency Responder Points:

- Sensory struggles may create a reaction to warm or cool rooms that is exaggerated. This could also include spaces such as an ambulance or police car.

   a. They may want to strip their clothing off if they feel extremely warm or become very restless and want to leave the space.

- It is incredibly important for first responders to understand that an autistic person may not react to pain in the way others do. Again, they may be over-responsive to pain or under responsive to pain.

   a. They may scream in pain at a touch that others would barely even notice, or they may not feel and have no reaction to a severe wound.
   b. Not reacting to a severe injury, combined with not being able to communicate their needs can be dangerous and certainly complicate treatment.
   c. They may also produce odd behaviors such as laughing, humming, singing, or removing clothing as a response to pain.

- The touch of a band aid or bandage may be upsetting to them; they might feel it more intensely than a neurotypical person would and may it elicit a strong negative reaction.
- It is often helpful to touch distal to proximal (start with further away and less invasive procedures and gradually move closer and more invasive) when examining and treating a person who shows touch sensitivity or is suspected of having struggles.

Presentation Topic – How are Social Skills Affected?

Material to be Presented:

Appropriate social interactions are important for a happy and productive life. Forging friendships and having good relationships with others is dependent on successful social interactions. Those with autism want to be around other people but because social situations rarely go well, they end up accepting being alone. It is well understood that autistic individuals experience social functioning challenges and it is also well understood that despite the challenges, people with autism desire social connection. It is not about a lack of interest in a social life, it's about understanding how to navigate a social system that the neurotypical population learns and establishes with a mutual understanding that is not a naturalistic process for autistic individuals. Those with ASD may exhibit social difficulties in a variety of areas and nuances.

- They may have difficulty making and maintaining eye contact/gaze or looking someone in the eyes or facial area.

   a. The problems with eye contact could be due to sensory seeking or avoiding. They may exhibit too much eye contact or too little.
   b. Many people with ASD report eye contact makes them dizzy and they cannot concentrate on anything else if they look in the speaker's eyes.
   c. One teenage boy likes to get very close and stare deeply into people's eyes as he greets them which can make the other person uncomfortable.
   d. A military man taught his son, who has autism, "Look 'em in the eye, Son!" whereupon the child learned to lock eyes with the listener, which would become quite disconcerting after a period of time.
   e. An autistic child has a process of turning all the family pictures and figurines backward so as not to see the faces.

- They may have an inability to interpret facial expression or other gestures. Understanding others' body language and displaying their own appropriate body language can be a challenge.

   a. After learning to interpret facial expressions, one girl would tell the others in her class, "Look at Teacher's face! Her face says, 'You're wrong!'"
   b. A man tells a story of attending a ballgame with his brother and nephew who has ASD. The young boy kept asking for nachos, and his father, interested in the action on the field, kept nodding and pointing to the nachos on the dad's lap. This was the dad's way of indicating to the child that Dad wished to share the nachos with the family. The child did not understand the nod or the pointing and did not realize he could have some of the nachos until it was verbalized.
   c. When the individual sees an angry person, they may laugh, because the red face, the squinty eyes, and the pursed lips look funny and they do not understand this is an angry communication.

- They may have poor social and/or emotional connections.

    a.   Infants and toddlers with autism may not respond to voices, or to attempts to play pat-a cake, peek-a-boo, etc. Often parents of autistic children will report not feeling connected to their child.

- They may have little or no interest in others, especially by neurotypical standards of interaction and relationship.

    a.   They may want to play with others, but not understand how to engage socially and relationally. Also, they may not need the same level and affirmation of being connected that neurotypical individuals require.

- They often lack the ability to see things from another's point of view or perspective.

    a.   This is often called "mind blindness" or theory of mind deficits. It affects the ability to understand turn-taking, that someone can have a different opinion, and expressions of kindness and comfort to others.

    b.   When Alex attended the Christmas party at City Hall, he noticed other small children playing and dancing at the Christmas tree. When his parents encouraged him to join in the fun, he soon returned in tears, claiming the other children were laughing at him. His mother attempted to explain they were laughing because it was fun to dance and be a little wild and they were not in any way laughing at him. He could not be convinced.

- They may struggle with understanding various forms of humor and/or be inappropriate or have bad timing in their own humor attempts.
- They may be very literal and concrete in their thinking and struggle in social situations that are more abstract.
- They may exhibit an extreme attachment or obsession to a toy or object.

    a.   Ava was attached to acorns as a small child and had to carry some acorns with her everywhere she went.

    b.   Samuel was extremely attached to two bobby pins that had to be with him always – in his pocket wherever he went, in his bed at bedtime, and even laying on the tub beside him during bath time.

- They may play with toys in unusual or unexpected ways or want to play with objects that are not traditionally considered toys.

    a.   A typical child will play with a toy car by running it on an imaginary road. The child with autism may choose to simply spin the wheel or to visually examine the toy for long periods of time.

    b.   They may enjoy toys or activities normally associated with a much younger child. A large teenage boy was riding the little frog ride at the amusement park along with the toddlers. Although unorthodox play may be pleasing to the child, it can also create problematic social situations and lead to teasing and bullying.

- They may be afraid of things they do not need to fear (something irrational like a toilet flushing) and not fear things most people would be afraid of like walking into traffic.

  a. This can also apply to fearing or a lack of fear of people, which in some scenarios could be dangerous.
  b. When Jeremy was two years old, he fearlessly scampered up onto the roof of the family workshop building with no concern or awareness of falling.
  c. They may fear something such as butterflies or flies because of the unpredictable flight patterns they display.

- They may shun or crave physical contact with others.

  a. Physical contact of any type may make them uncomfortable or they may like physical contact but in their own way and on their own terms.

- They often need predictability and a routine; change is difficult and spontaneous happenings can often be dysregulating.

  a. They like routines and schedules because they need to know what to expect, this is comforting and regulating and helps prevent anxiety and behavior reactions.
  b. The therapist may understand the person's need for consistency and establish a routine for how the session will start and end, which will be followed each time the person attends a session.

- They may exhibit unusual actions or movements and do this repeatedly.

  a. This is often referred to as stimming and examples include spinning, flapping the arms, turning lights on and off, humming, and bouncing.
  b. Each time Ben saw his favorite teacher, he would start flapping his hands rapidly with excitement.

- They may seem to want to be alone or withdrawn and may require less social interaction than neurotypical individuals. They may also require alone time to help regulate their system as social interactions can often be draining.
- They may have a hard time interacting with others even on a basic level. Social encounters may be extremely anxiety producing and there may be a lack of understating in how to navigate and keep social interactions flowing.

- They may have strong behavior reactions (outbursts) in social situations. This could be due to a lack of social skills, sensory struggles, or communicative struggles

Educator Points:

- Autistic children are often not socially motivated. Unlike neurotypical children, they are not rewarded by hearing, "Good job," seeing the teacher smiling and nodding, or by the promise of a rewarding play time with the other students. Their motivation to complete school work is often due to a desire to finish the task and be left alone, a desire to follow the rules (do what is expected), or because it taps into a special interest or obsession.
- They can be rule followers to the extreme. They may get agitated if others are not following established rules and struggle with flexible, ambiguous, and informal rules.

   a. One child was upset because the teacher was reading aloud in the library and the rule is "be quiet in the library."
   b. Children may get upset about a change in the rules or an adjustment in the schedule, for example, changes due to a fire drill. One student became distressed because the rule was to go to PE class at 9:30, but there was a fire drill at that time, and they could not meet that schedule.

Presentation Topic – What Behaviors May be Associated with ASD?

Material to be Presented:

Although characteristics vary widely from person to person with ASD, there are some thoughts on behavior that can be considered more uniform across the spectrum. First, behavior is an attempt to communicate, it is understood as communication when other forms of communication may not be expressible. Second, a person's behaviors are their way of telling others they have a need, a sensory overload, and/or a frustration. Lastly, unwanted behavior is not premeditated, planned, or a type of thought-out manipulation. It is a reaction and should be understood as an important tool for better understanding and helping the autistic person. There can exist multiple behaviors that may be observed in people with autism.

Key Points:

- Behaviors are typically the person with autism's way of communicating when other methods of communication are not viable. They are communicating something through the behavior that needs to be seen, heard, and understood.

- A dysregulated meltdown is not the same as a temper tantrum. It is a state of being where a person has become overwhelmed with an inability to control their emotions and reactions. It is not premeditated and is usually an upsetting experience for the individual.

Talking Points:

- They may withdraw and isolate themselves.
- They may display aggression due to problems in communication and frustrations about sensory input, anxiety, or confusion they receive from the environment.
- They could display self-stimulation such as rocking, jumping, flapping the hands, humming, or chanting.
- They will typically exhibit dysregulated meltdowns as opposed to temper tantrums.
- They may have an unusual pattern of interests, such as a high interest in one topic, like dinosaurs, vacuums, fans, or the solar system.
- They might desire order, "sameness," and extreme organization.

    a.   Parents described a child who liked to put things in a line. He even enjoyed straightening the cans on the shelves in the grocery store.

- They may have a preoccupation with certain behaviors and display odd routines or rituals.

    a.   A person may have rituals such as flipping the lights on and off repeatedly or refusing to go through certain doorways.
    b.   Charlie would hold his breath and duck quickly through a doorway to avoid getting the previous person's "stuff" on him.

- They might possess unusual mannerisms and appear somewhat "off" to others.
- They may lack appropriate response to pain.
- They could laugh inappropriately and not display socially accepted responses.
- They often exhibit odd or repetitive play that others may not recognize as play.
- They may be uncomfortable with the physical presence of others and/ or touch.
- They often have difficulty in regulating their emotions, usually challenges in identifying and expressing emotions accurately.
- They may be drawn to water without appropriate caution. This is especially true when wandering or running away.

Educator Points:

- Try to understand what motivates each child. This will likely be different for each autistic child and may be something unique and nontraditional.
- Children with ASD are not typically socially motivated. Do not place neurotypical motivation standards on autistic children and expect the process to be beneficial.
- When there is a behavior incident, observe what happened before, during, and after the behavior incident. Do not assume the child is being manipulative. It might be beneficial to complete a behavior assessment such as the Questions About Behavior Function (QABF) inventory which can be accessed online.

Emergency Responder Points:

- Using the information provided by the 911 dispatcher and/or the caregiver, be flexible and prepared to modify an approach as needed to best help the autistic person. Be prepared for unexpected reactions to sensory stimuli and approach situations with calmness and patience.
- It may be comforting to an agitated patient to wrap them in a blanket. They may resist any type of rescue activity and have a heightened sense of anxiety and confusion about what is happening and what the emergency responder is trying to do.
- It may be helpful to demonstrate each action on another person so the individual with ASD understands what will be happening and what will be expected of them.
- As mentioned previously, it is often helpful to perform the exam in a distal to proximal manner – start with further away and less invasive procedures and gradually move closer and become more involved.
- During an exam, be aware of the possibility of positional asphyxia as many people with ASD have poor core body strength.

Presentation Topic – Why is Autism Called a Spectrum Disorder?

Material to be Presented:

The Autism Society of America (2020) defined autism by a certain set of behaviors and as a "spectrum condition" that affects individuals differently and to varying degrees. Autistic individuals may have some similar unifying problem areas, but the severity of their difficulty and the presence or absence of other features will vary, such as fine motor ability, intelligence, increased or decreased verbal output, and social strengths (Coplan, 2010).

Autism is a spectrum disorder meaning there are many manifestations and ways a person could be affected by autism.

Key Points:

- Do not assume because you are familiar with one person with autism that all those with autism will look or act the same and have the same strengths and deficits as the person you are familiar with.
- Discover how each person with ASD is affected by their autism and view each as an individual who's autism manifests in specific and unique ways.
- Do not assume, stereotype, or stigmatize based on some notion or limited experience with autism.

Presentation Topic – How is Autism Diagnosed?

Material to be Presented:

Diagnosis of autism is typically given through a thorough psychological evaluation conducted by a trained psychologist which would be a medical diagnosis. Schools may also implement testing to diagnose for ASD which would be an educational diagnosis. Psychiatrists, neurologists, and medical doctors are also capable of providing a medical ASD diagnosis. The most thorough, unbiased, and quantitative process for diagnosing ASD is having the person participate in a psychological evaluation. This process typically includes several assessment/evaluation inventories and the process can take anywhere from 3 hours to two days to complete (Grant, 2018a).

Key Points:

- It is considered that a reliable and accurate diagnosis of ASD can be acquired as early as 18 months of age.
- Many autistic individuals do not receive a diagnosis at 18 months of age; most diagnosis of ASD occurs between the ages of 4.5 and 5.5.
- The earlier the diagnosis, the earlier needed therapies can begin, and early intervention with ASD has produced the best research outcomes for gains in skill and functioning ability.

Presentation Topic – What Causes Autism?

Material to be Presented:

There are many theories as to the cause of autism and why it is increasing at such a fast rate. It is suspected that there may be a genetic factor and an environmental factor involved, although no cause has been proven. The important awareness is to know that a parent's behavior does not cause autism. Theories about autism being caused by emotionally cold parents have long been disproven. Claims are made on almost a daily basis of various causes and links to autism, but currently there is no known cause – only multiple theories.

Key Points:

- Some autistic individuals or parents of children with autism may have very strong opinions about what causes autism.
- With no one theory being clearly conclusive, it seems reasonable to assume that some of the causes of autism, and increasing rates of diagnoses, are a result of multiple or a combination of factors.
- These factors may include abnormalities in brain structure or function; genetic influences; problems during pregnancy or delivery; and environmental factors such as viral infections, metabolic imbalances, and exposure to chemicals.

Presentation Topic – How is Physical Contact Affected?

Material to be Presented:

As Figure 7.14 illustrates, autistic individuals may crave or avoid physical contact with others. The touch from another person might be painful when the sense of touch is overly developed. There are others who are perfectly fine with having someone touch them, especially if they are the one to initiate the physical contact. Sometimes a stronger, firm touch is more easily accepted than a light, feathery touch, and other times both may feel painful. Some with autism may crave physical contact and rush to hug or grab another person, even a stranger.

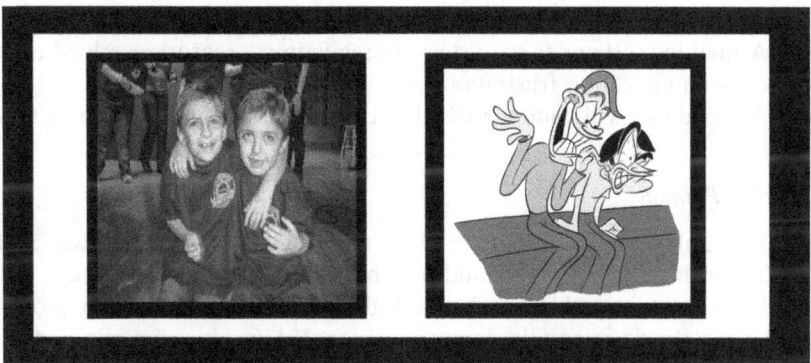

Figure 7.14 Those with ASD may crave or shun physical contact
Source: Photo courtesy of E. Obrey; Illustration courtesy of Landon Kemp

Key Points:

- Observe and ask those with ASD how they feel about physical contact. Ask them how much space they prefer and how touch feels to them.
- Do not assume that an autistic person is rude because they do not shake hands or engage in a hug.
- Try to respect the physical space and contact preferences of those with ASD.

Presentation Topic – Is a Meltdown Just a Temper Tantrum?

Material to be Presented:

A meltdown is different from a tantrum. Temper tantrums are thrown by a person who wants something, such as a toy, or wants to avoid something, such as chores. When they get what they want, the tantrum ends. They rely on having an audience, and normally will not continue the tantrum otherwise. A meltdown, on the other hand, is a result of the person's system becoming dysregulated, overwhelmed, or overstressed. Meltdowns are based on sensory overload or total communicative frustration. This does not end by reaching a goal, but more likely ends by fatigue and the individual calming over time. A meltdown is not dependent on having an audience. The person may truly need help to regain control. While a temper tantrum normally lasts a few minutes, a meltdown can continue for several hours. A tantrum requires an audience, while a meltdown will proceed even if no one is paying attention to the person.

Key Points:

- A tantrum stems from a person wanting something or wanting to avoid something. It is often goal directed and manipulative.
- A tantrum requires an audience for the behavior to continue.
- A tantrum subsides when the person achieves their goal.
- A meltdown stems from system dysregulation - sensory overload and/ or communication frustration.
- A meltdown will continue whether the person has an audience or not.

Talking Points:

- Remember that parents have likely experienced many meltdowns and know their child the best and how best to manage a meltdown.
- While it is acceptable to calmly ask the parent if they need help, professionals should respect the parent's decision. If a parent communicates they have the situation under control, allow the parent to work through the meltdown without interfering.
- Do not make judgmental comments or give disapproving looks.

- If there is a quiet area where a parent can take a child while they manage through a dysregulated meltdown, offer that to the parent.
  a. Hollie says Liam's meltdowns can last all day, until he is utterly exhausted, then the meltdown ends.
  b. Sarah says Olivia's meltdowns could last over four hours and nothing seems to help resolve them.
  c. One mother described it this way, "My neighbor's son cried for 15 minutes because he wanted candy in the checkout line. My child screamed for four hours because he heard water running."

Presentation Topic – What is Asperger's Syndrome?

Material to be Presented:

Asperger's syndrome is technically one form of autism, often characterized by sensory and social challenges. People with Asperger's syndrome usually have difficulties with social situations but not with language development. They are often very literal thinkers and struggle to understand humor, figures of speech, sarcasm, and words with multiple meanings. They may be rigid in their schedules, and often have sensory issues. Those with Asperger's usually function well in daily life and in society even though they struggle with social expectations and understanding. Cognitive abilities can range from average intelligence to gifted in those with Asperger's.

Key Points:

- The current version of the Diagnostic and Statistical Manual (DSM) which is used to diagnose autism, categorizes all autism as autism spectrum disorder. Prior to the current version, the DSM described three separate diagnoses that fell under the autism spectrum – autistic disorder, Asperger's syndrome, and pervasive developmental disorder.
- Even though the current DSM does not recognize Asperger's syndrome as a diagnosis, many individuals still use the term and identify as having Asperger's.

Presentation Topic – What to Tell People if They Suspect Their Child has Autism

Material to be Presented:

If a parent is questioning their child's behavior, a good place to start is advising them to talk to their pediatrician. They should make this contact as soon as possible. Their doctor can give them the information needed to contact services for evaluation, diagnosis, and treatment. A helpful book to suggest is *Stars in Her Eyes; Navigating the Maze of Childhood Autism* (Barboa & Obrey 2017). This book will guide them through the diagnosis process and into intervention decisions. It is important to provide assurances to parents who may fear a possible autism diagnosis, as it can be the key to unlocking many doors, such as educational services and financial assistance. It is also helpful for parents to talk to others who have an autistic child, as those individuals can share personal experiences and provide information about resources and services.

Presentation Topic – Future Expectations

Material to be Presented:

Individuals who are more mildly impaired regarding their autism are likely to be successful in college and excel in the fields of science and medicine. Traits commonly noted in people with autism such as a strong need for structure and intense focus on interests, can be an asset in the workforce in many different fields. Adaptations and modifications may be needed along with special training for both the individual and the employer. Although they may need some assistance, most people who are less impaired can become independent, contributing members of society. Those who have a more severe impairment may not be able to work or may require a job coach. They may not be able to live independently and may require assistance with living skills.

Key Points:

- Autistic adults often have some special needs or issues they must navigate. Each person's needs will differ, and what they may or may not need assistance with will vary.
- Some may access vocational training to help identify their strengths and interests.
- Some may acquire job opportunities where the employer and co-workers have been trained to understand the challenges of autism.
- Some individuals may live in group homes, supervised apartments, or other alternate living arrangements.
- Some may need help finding recreational and social opportunities where they can feel accepted and not judged.

Talking Points:

- Autism involves continuous, lifelong progress in many areas, including social awareness, learning new skills, and finding new enjoyable experiences.
- What do autistic adults need to be successful? They need compassionate, continuous support in areas neurotypical individuals may take for granted.

- They need understanding from the community as they try to lead fulfilling lives.
- Each adult with autism will look differently in terms of how they are navigating their life. Professionals should meet each person where they are and be willing to provide helpful guidance and support.

Presentation Topic – Many Faces, One Team

Summary to be Presented:

When raising any child, the typical responsibilities for care fall to the parent or guardian. Daily care involves nourishment, basic needs, and teaching activities of daily living. When daylight fades and the rest of the world goes to sleep, care for the child with ASD continues. The special needs of an autistic child continue around the clock with few to no breaks (Obrey & Barboa, 2015).

As the autistic child's world expands to include extended family members, everyone involved must learn new concepts and new skills to make relationships work. Becoming involved in school, religious groups, and other activities adds yet another dimension to family life. This increases the community of people who must be informed of the challenges and joys of experiencing a child with autism. The makeup of a community including retail, restaurants, first responders, medical personnel, and civic organizations can be pivotal in providing services to children and families, but education for how to best serve people and families affected by ASD is critical.

While there is a wealth of information that pertains to addressing the general population, there must be strategies pertinent and helpful for the autism and special needs populations. When professionals (individuals and organizations) make a commitment to absorb basic knowledge about ASD, and apply that knowledge to focused strategies for helping those with autism and special needs, all people associated with a child can become part of a nurturing cohesive team to allow the child the best life possible. This is the goal of the *Autism Friendly Training Program* and the benefits that can come from professionals committing to be autism friendly.

Autism Friendly means being aware of communication, social, and environmental factors that might impact people with ASD. It means looking for possible ways to modify the communication methods and the physical environment to better meet each individual's special needs. It also means trying to understand the processing, reacting, and responding differences a person with autism may have and ultimately, it means being friendly (patient, kind, and willing to try).

Bonus Presentation Topic: Helping Children Understand Autism

Material to be Presented:

This material covers a special presentation outline designed to help children become autism friendly.

Introduction: (5 minutes)

Introduce the presenters and give this autism scenario:

> Today we are going to talk about autism and being a friend.
>
> When I was in school, I liked my teachers, I liked math and reading. But most of all I liked my friends. One day on the playground I saw a little girl waiting by the door holding her hands over her ears waiting for the bell to ring. I went to find out why she had her hands over her ears. She told me she has autism and explained that the bell is super loud to her. She was waiting by the door because she didn't like being in the running rush when the bell rang. I told her there was still time to play and I would walk with her when the bell rang. She became a very good friend and over time taught me a great deal about autism.
>
> Two things happened that day. I learned about autism and I made a new friend.

Senses: (5 minutes)

> Now we are going to talk about our senses.
> We use our senses to get information about the world.

Have all the children raise one hand. Instruct them to put their thumb next to their ear. Put one finger by their eye, nose, mouth, and chin. Explain how this represents their five primary senses. Engage the children in naming the senses.

> When kids have autism, their senses can be higher or lower than ours.
>
> Sometimes noises that do not bother the rest of us, like the air conditioner, hurt their ears. Other times they really like loud noises such as fire trucks. Sometimes sunlight is painful to their eyes. Other times they love to look at bright lights. Sometimes they love to smell lotion on other people. Sometimes they hate the smell of flowers. Sometimes they hate the taste of something, that other people might love. Sometimes they do not like to be touched at all. Other times they really want to hug.

Communication: (5 minutes)

Communication is the way we tell others what we are thinking about or what we are feeling or need.
Some kids with autism:

Do not talk
Use sign language
Use a tablet to talk

If they talk:

They may have a hard time continuing a conversation.
Usually are literal thinkers (may need to define literal thinking).
They may not understand jokes.

Some kids with autism talk too much or only want to talk about one thing like dinosaurs. It's OK to say, "My turn to talk" or "Let's talk about something else, like baseball today."

Introduce the book Albert is My Friend *by Barboa and Luck (5 minutes)*

We are going to read a book called Albert is My Friend. It is about Albert and Mary Louise.
Mary Louise is a sweet little girl.
Albert does not talk.
They are friends.
Mary Louise talks about some of Albert's unusual behaviors.
Albert thinks about why he has those behaviors.

Read Albert is My Friend *and Explain friendship: (5 minutes)*

Talk about how to be a friend.

If you see someone alone on the playground, introduce yourself and ask them if they want to play with you.
Ask them to join your group.
Make sure they understand the game you are playing.
In the classroom smile and say "Hello" to them in the morning.
Have your mom ask their mom for a play date.
Invite them to your birthday party.
Never leave anyone out when you play.

Talk about how we are all different: hair, eyes, skin, height, etc. and why it is important to accept differences and not reject children who are different from us.

Conclusion: (5 minutes)

Read this poem to the group.

> I am different and that's OK.
> I am different, and I like me that way.

Have the children repeat it.

Pick 3–5 children to be "helpers." Have the helpers stand and repeat the poem together for a third time.

> I am different and that's OK.
> I am different, and I like me that way.

Praise and thank the children for being a good audience and encourage them to use the strategies they have learned here today. You may even want to give each child a certificate indicating they learned about being autism friendly.

The outline and information provided in this chapter serves as a guide for those who would facilitate an *Autism Friendly Training*. It is important to understand the audience that will be receiving the information. Some audiences may be specific such as first responders while other audiences may be a collection of different professionals. The presenter will adapt the presentation to meet he needs of the attendees. The information provided here represents a great many helpful points to share but each presenter will modify the content as needed for the particular group in which they are presenting.

Those who wish to solidify becoming an autism friendly presenter would complete one or more of the *Autism Friendly Trainings* which can be found on the AutPlay® Therapy website – www.autplaytherapy.com. The training options include: The *Autism Friendly Training*, The *Autism Friendly Play Therapist* (for mental health professionals), *Autism Friendly Kids*, and The *Training the Presenter Training (To Become an Autism Friendly Presenter)*.

8 Being Autism Friendly

Information for Specific Groups

The *Autism Friendly Presentation* discussed in Chapter 7 provides information to meet the needs of anyone seeking general information about autism and serving autistic individuals. The chapter includes specific talking points for educators and first responders in addition to general information that can be applicable to anyone. Information was added in Chapter 7 specific to educators and first responders as these are the groups who have most often requested training about autism. While Chapter 7 addresses the general population and those two specific classifications of attendees, there will be times when other groups require specialized information. Chapter 8 presents information for several additional groups to consider in becoming autism friendly.

Grandparents and Other Extended Family Members

Becoming a grandparent, aunt, uncle, or cousin is one of life's greatest joys. Many families celebrate the arrival of a new addition to the family and the typical expectation is that the new member will be neurotypical. Some families quickly discover that the new child in the family is not neurotypical and has a diagnosis called autism. When a family is presented with a child with differing abilities, it is natural to wonder what lies ahead, experience uncertainties, and even deal with a level of grief.

A million questions may flood over the family when there is a child with ASD. Often it is the parent who is the major source of information and can help other family members better interact with the autistic child. They can share with the extended family members what calms the child, what they enjoy, and what special quirks or nuances the child may display. Family members will want to strive to be a source of help and support for both the parents and the child. Too often parents report that one of their primary stressors is extended family members who do not understand and may even devalue the child with autism. Information about ASD and the *Autism Friendly Training* presented in this book will be helpful for family members. In addition to the information provided here, family members can continue to seek out new and helpful information to continue their own growth in understanding and supporting autism.

DOI: 10.4324/9781003105633-9

Over time, family members will learn to understand and accept the strengths and weaknesses of the differently abled family member. Relatives will understand the schedule, adjustments, and processes that might revolve around the member with ASD. Some family activities and rituals will become quite routine and the autistic individual will soon understand what to expect from family members and what those family members expect from them. As the family navigates among other family members, it can be helpful explaining to the individual with ASD in simple terms what will happen and how they should act in different homes, around different family members, and at family events.

People with autism need to know what to expect and until this is well established, relatives might find it helpful to use the PrepChat© (Obrey & Barboa, 2015). A PrepChat© is a simplified short chat an adult has with an individual to give an upcoming situation some predictability. It tells the person what is going to happen as an event approaches. This may be something that is going to happen soon or in the distant future. The adult may repeat the preparation several times as the event approaches. For example, a PrepChat© could be used to teach the individual to ask a relative for help when they are at the relative's house:

> Sometimes things are hard.
> You try your best.
> Sometimes you can't do things by yourself.
> You can ask Grandma or Grandpa for help. We will help you when you ask us.

Another example would be using a PrepChat© to prepare an individual with ASD if they are going into a crowded store.

> Sometimes the store is crowded with a lot of people.
> It is kind to say "Excuse me" if people are in your way.
> You should say "Excuse me" to show you are nice.
> You should be patient and wait.
> If people hear you, they will let you through.

An additional example would be using a PrepChat© for improving a specific behavior such as yelling, running away, or hitting.

> Sometimes you yell.
> You can yell if you are playing some games.
> You can yell if it is an emergency.
> You don't yell if you are mad.
> You don't yell if everyone else is quiet.

People with autism often need to hear the same instructions given many times to learn the rules family members are teaching them. It is important to be patient. Over time the understanding will progress. Research shows that individuals with ASD need repetition to master new skills. As an individual's behaviors improve, family members can continue to make frequent use of the PrepChat© to prepare the person for additional situations and acquiring more skills.

An additional behavior strategy family members might employ is the ChoicesChat© (Obrey & Barboa, 2015). ChoicesChat© are short simple discussions an adult has with an autistic individual about a social problem that has occurred. If the person is functioning at a cognitive level where they can participate in a discussion, talking about choices that may have led up to a problem and what might be a better choice the next time can help the person improve behaviors. An example would be using a ChoicesChat© to address an incident that had happened.

GRANDPA: Why was Aiden hitting and crying?
CHILD: I took his cookie.
GRANDPA: Was that a good choice?
CHILD: No.
GRANDPA: Who was hurt?
CHILD: Aiden was mad because he didn't get a cookie.
GRANDPA: What did Grandpa have to do?
CHILD: You took my own cookie away.
GRANDPA: What would be a better choice next time?
CHILD: I should not take someone else's cookie.

Using a PrepChat© or ChoicesChat© requires the individual to have a level of understanding to engage and benefit from a discussion. These techniques are individualized to each situation and for each person. If a child is having trouble sharing with their cousins, the conversation should be built around that specific problem. The person does not need to be verbal to benefit from this technique. The point is to provide a tool for teaching social behavior in an easy to understand guideline. As an individual advances in their thinking, family members can modify the chats to meet the person's increasing level of understanding and their current social needs. When teaching through these strategies, family members should monitor their own emotional reactions and try to remain calm.

If a person is more impaired or still in early learning stages and cannot understand what they are being told, family members should coordinate with the parents. Be willing to listen to parents to find out what strategies they find helpful and useful and attempt to keep behavior management tools consistent across the environments. Being consistent from family member to family member and environment to environment will help the individual improve behavior more smoothly and quickly. If parents have a certain strategy or approach that is effective for the child, other family members should try to learn this approach and apply it when they are with the child.

Another tool that is helpful for extended family members is scheduling. Scheduling often helps a person with autism feel calm, regulated, and more organized. Individuals with ASD typically thrive with order and predictability; this is why they often line up objects. Schedules may be created by placing pictures in a line, allowing them to predict what will come next. The schedule may show all the activities in a day, or it may help the person complete one single task. If the individual can read, use written words in the schedule. If they cannot read, draw pictures, or print them from a computer and paste them onto the schedule. Using pictures of the real situations can also be helpful and there are several apps available on tablet devices that can be used to create visual schedules. An example would be a visual schedule with pictures of each of the steps needed to brush their teeth.

Grandparents and other family members can be helpful in teaching the autistic individual to relax and self-regulate. When a person can learn to calm themselves, it allows them some control over their behaviors. Helping the grandchild learn positive coping skills will alleviate many negative and/ or unwanted behaviors the child may display to cope with anxiety. Through trial and error, the family member might discover that giving the person a "stress ball" or a soft fidget toy helps the individual to calm. Or perhaps providing a quiet place in the home the autistic person can go and be by themself or access to a movement toy such as a mini trampoline or exercise ball can help the individual calm themself. If the family can reduce the external stimuli when the person is stressed (turn down the lights, lower the noise level), they may be able to calm themself more easily. The individual may be able to learn to use deep breathing or softly repeat a phrase such as, "It's OK, it's OK" to self-regulate. Many persons with ASD find it calming to wrap themselves in a blanket. If the individual has a weighted vest or other object that has been prescribed for them by an occupational therapist, ask the parent to send it with them when they come for a visit and learn how to use it correctly. It is critical to use the same strategies at the relative's house as the parent uses at home for teaching social skills and self-regulation.

School Support Staff

The support positions in schools carry a heavy responsibility, require extraordinary patience, and a dedicated spirit. Food service workers, secretaries, maintenance workers, librarians, bus drivers, duty teachers, nurses, paraprofessionals, and school resource officers all play an important part in our educational system. With the increase in prevalence of autism in our communities it is expected that school support staff will have contact with students with autism. Support staff deserve to have adequate preparation and the necessary tools to know what to expect from and how to serve autistic individuals. Each support professional, in their own way, will have a role in keeping children safe at school. This book and training program are not meant to supersede any school policy manual, but to offer suggestions to improve services to children with autism. School policies and procedures are the first line of protection and all staff must familiarize themselves with those documents and adhere to the standards. That being understood, all school support staff who have contact with students with ASD, should have access to the *Autism Friendly Training* highlighted in this book.

The first line of managing behaviors in any "non-classroom" area of the school is to focus on prevention of the problem. Remember that behavior is the child's way of communicating when they do not have the skills needed to express effectively or to cope with a problem. Expectations for bus riding, library, recess, the cafeteria, or other times outside the classroom should include a concrete discussion of the expectations and rules (preferably in a visual format). Autistic children are usually strong rule followers so this will be comforting to them and an important staff tool to prevent behavior issues.

A good example is bus drivers who have the responsibility of setting the tone for the day as the child enters the bus (their first contact with a school representative), and setting the tone for a happy family time once the child exits the bus to go home. The child's experience on the bus is highly important. Children with ASD depend on predictability. Knowing what to expect in each situation is essential for maintaining regulation; it comforts the child and helps them cope. The challenge for bus drivers is to give the child the predictability they need while at the same time navigating any changes that inevitably occur. It would be uncommon for a typical bus driver to have a working knowledge of autistic children without having acquired additional and specific training. Many bus drivers have a primary responsibility of driving the bus and not focusing on helping a child regulate. Yet, autistic children often need some additional consideration when riding a bus to and/or from school. Children with autism need to feel safe riding a bus and they need to know that the bus driver is a support person.

Preparation is key and will be a joint effort by the parent, the teacher, and the bus driver. Besides discussing the bus schedule and any possible changes to the timeline, the child should be taught actual bus riding skills. The child should be prepared for having to stand in a line. Patience and waiting are often not strengths for the child with autism and social rules regarding waiting in a line may not be understood. Showing them the rules on a visual chart made with pictures can be helpful. It's important to be certain each child knows the bus riding expectations. Do not assume they know a rule, just because it may seem like common sense does not mean that a child with ASD will automatically understand a rule. Make sure they know the bus driver and the bus aide are there to help them and it is the adult's job to keep them safe while they are on the bus.

Depending on the child's level of understanding, prepare them for possible emergencies and for any preparedness drills. Teach them that although there is a schedule, sometimes traffic is slow, or the road conditions may require a change in the schedule or route. Prepare for the bus riding experience by pre-assigning a seat for the student. On the bus, they may seem like an easy target for bullying by other students. To protect them from possible bullying, consider giving them a seat near the driver. If they will be sharing a seat, it will be helpful to make a visual seat divider, such as with tape displaying the section each person should be staying within. If the child carries a comfort item, allow them to bring it with them on the bus if it does not cause a safety risk.

Sensory overload and communication difficulties result in unwanted behaviors. The challenge is to reduce the sensory irritants and find ways to improve communication in order to ward off behavioral issues. Communication should be kept to a minimum, using clear, simple, concrete directions. Do not speak too fast. Pause for understanding as it may take them longer to process what is being said. The bus staff should be aware of stimuli that may cause a sensory problem. Be aware of the child's sensory issues and take an assessment of the bus they will be riding to make sure there are no sensory triggers. When a problem arises on a moving bus, this can be a safety issue for all the riders and the driver. The adults must be forward thinking and identify possible sources of agitation to prevent problems. The information highlighted for bus drivers could easily be interlaced for any school support person. The bus driver example highlights what most support staff in schools will need to consider, be trained on, and be prepared for when serving autistic children.

Cosmetologists and Barbers

As previously discussed, sensory integration is typically a major concern with autism. A person who has ASD may have very strong sensory reactions to many items in a salon or barber shop; even home-grooming can be a challenge. Due to possible visual confusions, a stylist attempting to serve a person with autism may find it helpful to approach them gently and explain what movements will be taking place. Preparing the individual before each action with clear simple explanations or a demonstration can help the process go more smoothly. Some persons may move or shake their head for sensory stimulation during the haircut. This is another reason to move more slowly and mindfully to avoid an accident. If the workstation is cluttered, this could be dysregulating and/or distracting to the autistic individual. Pictures may be helpful to explain to them the steps for their appointment; a visual display of what will happen in order from entering the shop to exiting. It may calm and distract them to let them play a video game on a tablet or watch a favorite video. Sometimes sucking or biting on a hard piece of candy can also help.

Cosmetologists may find it beneficial to move to a quieter station or area to reduce the client's agitation. Some autistic individuals may have sensory issues with noises in the salon or with certain materials such as a trimmer or a hair dryer. If the customer with autism does not respond to directives or questions, remember the background noise may be distracting them or preventing them from hearing the question. The worker will want to trouble shoot to help alleviate any issues such as if there is an extreme reaction to the sound of the water running, consider a waterless shampoo to avoid the behavior response. Or if there is an issue with mirrors, turn the person around so they cannot see into the mirror. For clients who are bothered by the sound of the clippers, allow them to wear ear plugs, earbuds, or use scissors instead of clippers. Others may actually prefer the sound of the clippers to the snipping of the scissors, so watch for signs of distress. Another issue may involve combs and brushes – a wide tooth comb or a pick may be more comfortable than a fine-tooth comb for some individuals.

Persons with problems in the vestibular sensory processing may have difficulty if the chair is raised to where their feet do not touch the ground. Many stylists use a weighted blanket to help the individual feel comfortable and safe. Another prevention/regulation strategy is for the stylist to allow the person to sit on the lap of a parent. It is important to explore alternatives to the specific sensory problems as they are identified. Stylists can learn to recognize the sights, sounds, smells, and touches that distress the client with ASD and implement alternative strategies. Stylists should spend some time creating a checklist of questions for autistic clients to better understand what their issues and preferences are and adjust the situation to meet their needs. Stylists should also spend time talking with the parents of a child with autism to better understand what can be done to make the appointment successful.

Restaurant Workers

Many individuals and families spend a considerable amount of time eating, meeting, and lounging in restaurants. This may be for meal planning, for entertainment, or for celebrations. According to Hamm (2020) the average American eats an average of 4.2 commercially prepared meals per week. In other words, on average, as a nation, Americans eat out between four and five times a week. This translates to just over 18 meals in an average month eaten outside the home. It is a common convenience that most families take for granted. Busy families may have all the adults in the home working full-time jobs, and eating out is a time and labor-saving alternative. Families plan dinners in restaurants as celebrations for family events, as part of entertainment experiences, for pragmatic reasons such as a meeting, and for fun. The reasons can vary but most families will experience a significant amount of time in restaurants.

For families with an individual with autism, that ease and convenience of going to a restaurant is often replaced with challenges, embarrassment, and rejection. The family planning a celebration may find themselves in a nightmare experience and regretting the choice to try a restaurant. A myriad of issues typically associated with autism can manifest to create an unhappy experience for the individual, the family, the restaurant staff, and the other patrons.

Restaurant workers have the ability to implement some simple modifications which can make the dining experience positive for all. If the family states they have a family member with autism or special needs, listen to them. If the family has suggestions that will make the dining experience go more smoothly, make an effort to follow their lead. If the family asks for a simple accommodation such as a certain way for the food to be prepared, make an effort to work with the family. If the parent requests a remote booth, or a table farther removed from other guests, it is helpful to make an effort to accommodate the request. If the parents request to pay earlier in the meal than normally expected, please allow them to pay the check. They may be preparing in case they need to leave abruptly.

When possible, accommodate slight tweaks in the food preparation or presentation. For example, they may ask to have the hamburger served on the side of the bun, rather than inside the bun. Understand that the person may be upset if the food does not look like what they expect. Be understanding if they reject the food due to it not looking how they expected. Allow food to be served in alternate presentations rather than the expected plate. Many persons with autism are much more comfortable having foods presented in small bowls, thereby preventing the various foods on the plate from touching the other foods.

Staff taking the food order should understand that it may take the autistic person longer to respond to questions. The processing of the question and the formation of the answer usually takes longer than would be typically expected. Be patient and do not rush the communication. Allow a little extra time for the customer to answer (Barboa & Luck, 2018a). Allow some flexibility in the charges for special orders that are no extra trouble. For example, if the person only wants a hot dog bun, do not charge them for the full hot dog combo meal that is listed on the menu. Avoid judgmental comments or disapproving looks. Be patient and understanding and pay attention to the information being given by the parents as this is key to preventing unwanted behavior and creating a calm, happy dining experience. Making simple accommodations such as these is the heart of being autism friendly.

Autism friendly educated restaurants are realizing that the possible ensuing meltdowns and unwanted behaviors from someone with ASD can be prevented and service can be pleasant for both the establishment and the family. It cannot be promised that by making autism friendly modifications a restaurant will completely prevent an unhappy, dysregulated person. However, with minor adjustments, staff understanding, and tweaking of routine procedures, many problems and meltdowns can be avoided. With a thoughtful, accommodating family service, the ASD family gains a quality dining experience and the restaurant has retained a happy customer, more likely to return to patronize the establishment.

Entertainment Workers

Entertainment venues of all types and sizes are focused on creating fun family experiences and building a customer base. Some examples of entertainment venues include movie theaters, fairs, museums, theme parks, zoos, video game centers, and kid play places. By following the suggestions in the general *Autism Friendly Training* program, these businesses can identify sensory, social, and communication issues in their environments and create alternatives to allow enjoyment for families affected by autism. Many families dealing with autism would enjoy participating in a variety of entertainment-based experiences but often shy away from such activities due to the myriad of possible issues that could be challenging for their autistic child.

A large entertainment venue located in Missouri is known for being a loud, stimulated, busy place where families come to have fun together. The entertainment center became aware that many families cannot participate in the fun due to having a family member with sensory processing issues. They decided to answer the call to action and remedy this situation. They partnered with the local Arc organization to learn how to make their venue sensory friendly. They organized a feasibility study to determine whether such an endeavor was even possible in such a loud, fun filled place. They established what they called a "Buddies" time, when the complex would open specifically for those affected by sensory challenges. Their accommodations included lowering the volume of the games by 60% and eliminating the abrasive lights and lighting patterns wherever possible. They provided use of noise-canceling headphones free of charge, and sunglasses to dim the lights that they could not modify. In areas that could not be minimized, they warned the families with signs that said, "louder zone." They provided informational handouts and updated their website to inform the parents of the layout, and what to expect if they were to attend a "Buddies" event.

During the regularly scheduled "Buddies" events, a complimentary pass was given to caregivers joining an individual who had come to participate. Rather than charge for each game separately at this time, there was a charge for the person to enter the play zone, with unlimited game access. They made this modification because some individuals have a very short attention span and move quickly from one game to the next, never really playing a game to completion. Activities such as the trampoline sessions were limited and only one person at a time was allowed to jump. The management turned off the deck lights on the go-carts and replaced the loud buzzer with spoken announcements indicating the end of the race. In the laser tag area, the venue offered some games with lights off, while others had lights on. In the XD motion theater, they alternated a sensory sensitive showing with a full sensory showing. Strobe lights were turned off and curtains were partially closed to dim the light. Motion chairs were modified for the sessions. Each feature/activity was assessed and modified as needed.

The Arc provided customized educational and training workshops for what evolved into the "Buddy Squad." Besides information about autism and other challenges, they learned how to encourage, support, and assist autistic children. They also learned what to do to prevent problems, including redirecting and supporting techniques. Through education, the employees became comfortable with possible behaviors they might see, and what to do if a person was having a crisis. They learned how to be comfortable with their own feelings, apprehensions, questions, and concerns. When the program came to fruition, they knew they had accomplished something utterly amazing. The comments made to the business by the many families who attended as well as online feedback, showcased how successful the "Buddies" program was and what a strong need there is for more programs such as this one.

Another autism friendly example is a national movie theater chain that has excelled in creating sensory movie sessions "for all." One afternoon a week the company adjusts their typical process and creates accommodations to better serve their sensory sensitive customers. Some of the adjustment include:

- lights are turned up and the sound is turned down,
- all ages are welcome (including infants),
- talking and noise is allowed, and guests can move around,
- latecomers are admitted,
- and adaptive technology is welcome (but no other electronics).

Some theatres are equipped with accommodations such as closed captioning devices, headsets for amplification, and descriptive audio. The University of California, Berkeley Web Access (2020) gives the following definitions of these technologies:

> "Descriptive audio" means that [the movie being shown] has additional audio content that describes aspects of the video that are purely visual and not accessible to blind or visually-impaired people. Usually, there's a second audio track that contains the description. Viewers can listen to the second track along with the primary track.

Captions are different – they're necessary to make audio content accessible to hearing-impaired people, and are also useful in situations where audio cannot be played. . .

Sometimes descriptive audio might be called "audio description" or "video description."

AMC Theatres have been running "sensory friendly films" since 2008, a program that now encompasses 175 locations. During movie time, the lights remain on and the sound is turned down and patrons are free to wander around the theater (Swetlitz, 2017). Sports stadiums across the country are also beginning to recognize the need to be autism friendly. One feature commonly employed is a sensory inclusive room available to fans. Families are welcome to use the quiet place away from the roaring crowd. These rooms are often equipped with toys and other items to relieve stress. These autism friendly rooms often feature low lights, bean bag chairs, and ear plugs among other accommodations.

Theme parks are beginning to include trainings for autism awareness. Parks, museums, and other attractions can implement simple changes such as providing a written guide telling about specific challenges that persons with autism may experience on various attractions. Parks and other entertainment venues may consider special access passes to avoid the long waits, and special viewing areas for some attractions. Entertainment venues may also consider a "Rider Switch" program that reduces time waiting in line (Allen, 2019).

According to a study conducted by the International Board of Credentialing and Continuing Education Standards (IBCCES), 87% of families with children with ASD do not go on family vacations (Allen, 2019). With completion of the *Autism Friendly Training Program* described in this book, venues can identify sensory, social, and communication challenges facing their customers. With even minor accommodations, these physical and social challenges can be addressed to enhance the entertainment experience for all families.

Retailer Workers

The amount of time and money the average family spends shopping is staggering. It is more than a necessity in modern days; it is a major source of recreation and enjoyment. According to Becker (2020), the average person makes 301 trips to stores annually, spending 400 hours a year in this activity. More than one-third of shoppers surveyed reported that shopping lifted their mood and was a source of pleasure. This information is based on neurotypical individuals and is not usually the experience for many families of neurodiverse individuals.

A trip to the store, with bright lights, music, shopping carts clanking, people moving swiftly in many directions, cash registers ringing, people talking, smells emanating from cosmetics or foods, and temperature changes throughout the store, can be terrifying to an individual with autism. For a person with sensory issues, trying on clothes or shoes may be excruciating. Others may feel a compulsion to feel every item in the store as they shop, or to straighten the items on the shelves. The individual may become upset when there are changes in the store, or when items are not in stock. A sensory overload can trigger behavioral challenges and meltdowns, thereby creating an unpleasant shopping experience for the family as well as for other shoppers.

As society becomes more aware of the sensory and regulation challenges of autism, some stores are instituting sensory free hours as a shopping option. On either a daily or weekly basis, they provide a quieter shopping time, with dimmer lights and less activity. The stores make an effort to reduce public address announcements during this time. Other establishments offer a quiet area where families can go to calm down if needed. Turner (2020) suggested that this could be an empty dressing room, or an out-of-the-way corner of the store. A large national chain store that recently completed and *Autism Friendly Training* reported they have become aware of some of their autistic customers and have been able to accommodate many needs. For example, one autistic customer would become visibly upset if their favorite candy was not in stock. The manager recognized their discomfort and asked them to be a special assistant and let the manager know if the candy is out of stock so it can be re-ordered. The man was happy with this special assignment and the manager now has a happy customer. At the same store, the manager noticed that a child felt a compulsion to feel or squeeze each item in the store, resulting in parental frustration as the mom tried to stop the behavior so they could complete their shopping. The manager offered the family the use of a squeeze ball to occupy the child as they shopped, which they could obtain from and return to the cashier. The parent was impressed and bragged on social media about the friendly store, recommending it to her friends.

Another strategy that can be used to improve the family shopping experience is the creation of an impulse limited checkout lane – a special checkout lane that has no "last minute" items for sale. If the parent can hurry through a checkout lane with no candy or small tempting impulse items on display, the whole trip may be more successful. If a store can implement a strategy to prevent a behavioral problem, this is always preferable to trying to calm an upset person once a meltdown has begun.

Sometimes children slip away and get lost in a large store. In these instances, an announcement is usually made, and the staff does a quick search of the shopping floor, calling out the name and locating the child. A staff that has completed the *Autism Friendly Training* will know they should search for an autistic child in a different way than when looking for a neurotypical child. Information from the parent can give the staff a quick clue as to whether the child would be trying to *avoid* sensory input or may be *seeking* sensory input. The staff could hurry to an isolated quiet hiding place or can check a place that may attract the specific child. As has been discussed for other considerations, the parent is the key to information about their child and retail workers should defer to parent-provided information.

In the event that an individual would have a sensory meltdown in a store, the best plan for the retail worker would be to follow the lead of the parent or the caregiver who is with the person and ask the caregiver how they could assist. The worker should not try to take over or solve the problem for the parent. The worker can do crowd control, tend to other children, assure a clear space for the parent to attend to the individual, and keep others from interfering and making the situation worse. When the behavior is under control, the parent might appreciate assistance in getting their items quickly checked out and taken to the car.

A recent study showed that 29% of shoppers would switch to another store to find an autism friendly retailer (Turner, 2020). By being autism friendly and learning to meet the customer's needs, retailers can retain loyal customers. When the staff of a store is trained to recognize sights, sounds, smells, or other sources of sensory overloads in the store, they can improve the quality of the shopping experience for families. This benefits the customer as well as the retailer. The customer will recognize the establishment cares about being autism friendly and typically return and bring friends.

Medical Professionals

A study of over 3,000 pediatricians and family practice physicians reported a widespread self-perceived lack of skills when working with those with autism (Golnik et al., 2009). This is disturbing considering that families affected by autism are likely to spend a large amount of time visiting medical professions. Some parents report being concurrently involved with an average of 4–5 different professionals and having 3–5 different appointments to attend each week. It is imperative that medical professionals are trained and feel competent working with those with ASD. Many in the medical community have found the first responders' section of the *Autism Friendly Training* to be helpful and applicable.

Medical professionals should be well-informed about ASD and the common comorbidities associated with the diagnosis. The National Alliance on Mental Illness (NAMI, 2020) listed the following commonly associated disorders:

- *Intellectual impairment* – The amount and type of cognitive challenge varies widely among people with ASD. Language skills or executive function may be weak. The medical professional must recognize possible communication barriers, such as inability to report pain, difficulty following directions, and struggles with answering questions. The professional must be prepared to allow extra time for a response when asking a question.

- *Seizures* – NAMI reports that one in four children with ASD has seizures of varying intensity.
- *Fragile X Syndrome* – According to NAMI, about 1 in 25 children with ASD have this gene mutation. This may complicate intellectual development.
- *Tuberous Sclerosis* – This gene mutation, although rare, should be considered by the professionals involved with the individual. This disorder has been linked to epilepsy and other health impairments.
- *Gastrointestinal problems* – Persons with autism report a high incidence of gastrointestinal discomforts, such as stomach pain, reflux, bowel problems, vomiting, and bloating.
- *Mental health conditions* – Anxiety disorders can develop in children and adults with ASD. There is also a correlation to Attention Deficit Hyperactivity Disorder (ADHD) and depression. Self-regulation is a common complaint, and it may fall to the mental health professional to help the family with this skill deficit. Caregivers of persons with high intensity meltdowns often turn to mental health professionals for help.

When discussing areas of stress, parents often cite difficulty finding medical professionals who are "autism savvy." Many parents feel that medical professionals are not aware of autism and do not understand how autism affects individuals. Further, they report that medical professionals do not listen to them and can often make things worse. A few easy accommodations can make a trip to a medical or dental office positive and more autism friendly. The professional should ask the parents to come prepared with written information about their autistic child and any questions they have. That way, at the appointment, information can be provided, and nothing is missed. If the appointment is to discuss a parental concern about the child's behavior, it may be helpful for the professional to ask the parent to provide video examples of the behaviors they are describing.

Medical doctors, dentists, and other professionals can learn to be aware of the sensory, social, and communicative challenges that add to the patient's anxiety. Visits to a new clinic, new doctors, and unfamiliar procedures and touches can greatly add to the discomfort for the autisitc individual. The newness of the environment adds to the patient's anxiety. Unfamiliar places and people usually increase anxiety and dysregulation for those with autism. Sensory stresses make visiting various medical professionals or a dentist highly stressful. In fact, many of the procedures that would typically accompany a visit to a medical professional are going to feel invasive and uncomfortable for those with ASD. Professionals should be mindful to provide services in the most calming and tranquil environment possible.

A common suggestion for medical professionals such as doctors and dentists involves the scheduling of appointments. This begins with appointment considerations. If the doctor's office is aware the person they are serving has autism, the office can consider scheduling this family during the slowest point of a busy day. Sitting for long periods in the waiting room can increase dysregulation and lead to a behavior outburst. The office should try to allow the family to remain in their car and call them when the doctor/dentist is ready to see them.

Communication can be essential for a more successful visit. Medical professionals should prepare parents for what to expect. The caregiver can in turn prepare the individual. Often, mental health professionals will create a social story to send to the individual before their first appointment. This short story describes what the person can expect on their first visit. Parents are instructed to read the story to their child several times before their first appointment. During a visit, the doctor, dentist, or other professional should describe to the patient what will happen each step of the procedure. A suggested strategy is to demonstrate any procedure on the doctor, nurse, or the parent so the person can see what will happen. For example, if an individual sees that the small dental mirror can easily be placed in the mouth to give a view of the back teeth, they may be more likely to calmly allow it. Another suggestion is for the medical professional to provide a comforting item such as a weighted blanket or vest for use during the visit. Many successful doctors and dentists provide a fun distraction to the client to take their mind off the fear of the unknown. The time taken to build a trusting relationship will be beneficial in providing a positive experience for the individual. At times, the medical doctor or dentist may have to think outside the box to discover nonstandard ways to implement needed medical procedures.

Along with medical professionals, individuals with autism often require the services of mental health professionals. Emotional and behavioral problems can be major issues for autistic people. Additionally, those with autism can suffer from trauma issues, attachment disorders, depression, poor self-worth, bullying, life adjustment challenges and a whole host of mental health related problems. As ASD is a mental health diagnosis, many mental health professionals are familiar with autism but many still lack training in how to effectively work with autistic individuals. Professionals should explore additional training such as the AutPlay® Therapy Certification Training (Grant, 2017a) designed for mental health professionals to increase their knowledge in working with individuals and families affected by autism.

Galanopoulos et al., (2014), described the following disorders that may be a focus for mental health professionals serving people with autism:

- *Anxiety disorders*: Approximately 40% of people with ASD have symptoms of an anxiety disorder, compared to 15% of the general population. Anxiety in turn can lead to depression. Communication problems may make it more difficult for the patient to describe the symptoms they are feeling. After forming a strong relationship with the individual, the mental health professional can work on anxiety reduction, acceptance, and desensitization.

- *Obsessive Compulsive Disorder (OCD)*: One particularly dominant anxiety disorder is OCD. A person with OCD has repetitive thoughts and behaviors that are upsetting to them. The mental health professional will address both the obsession and the compulsion. As OCD is under-recognized and under-treated, the mental health practitioner must be alert to the behavior signs. The professional must be knowledgeable about the behavioral and pharmaceutical options for treatment.
- *Depression*: As people with autism have difficulties in communication, identification of some problems, such as depression, may be difficult. Mental health professionals must know that persons with autism often have trouble labeling, describing, and sharing their feelings and emotions. Galanopoulos et al. (2014) stated that the person with ASD may find it hard to seek mental health assistance because they find change difficult. Transitions are anxiety-producing, and they may worry they have done something wrong and others will judge them.

Although autism is multi-faceted and complex, it is the observable behaviors that are usually the source of referrals to mental health professionals. Medical professionals may find it beneficial to refer a client to a mental health professional to address specific mental health challenges. Medical professionals should work collaboratively with mental health professionals and any other professionals who are involved with the individual and the family. A multifaceted collaborative approach to care is not unusual for autistic individuals and often results in the best treatment outcomes.

Churches and Other Places of Worship

Barboa and Allen (2018) stated that some of the most heartbreaking stories within the neurodevelopmental community relate experiences of families not being accepted by churches due to having a family member with autism. Many families continually search for an autism friendly church, going from one to another in hopes the next one will be accepting, while other families give up and no longer seek a place to worship, feeling it is a lost effort.

Committing to being an autism friendly church can have several different looks. One example would be to create a special needs ministry for those with autism which would begin with the selection of a team leader to navigate this process. The person in charge would assemble a leadership team, arrange training for the team and the congregants in general, and work with the church leadership to establish what is needed and feasible. Specialty committees can be formed to design program intake forms, welcome families, facilitate trainings, and develop outreach services for families with ASD and special needs. The leadership team can explore the ways the church can minister to autism families.

Barboa and Allen (2018) described the process for a church or other place of worship to implement a disability ministry which would involve key players such as a training coordinator, an event coordinator, a prayer coordinator, a secretary, and children's teachers. Many places of worship employ a buddy system. The buddy is paired with a person in need of a role model. The buddy might accompany their partner to services, help meet the individual's needs, encourage their friend, and assist in self-help skills, such as mobility, seating, playing games, eating, or toileting needs.

Additional initiatives include designing facility classrooms to be physically accessible and welcoming. Barboa and Allen (2018) suggested providing quiet areas within the classrooms. These areas will have less light and less noise. Special care must be taken to care for children who are a flight risk and may run out of a room. Two-way radios or the use of the parents' cell phones in case an issue arises is also a good strategy.

Restrooms should be wheelchair accessible with changing tables available for both children and adults. Many autistic individuals are terrified of hand dryers, so paper towels are preferred. Self-flushing toilets are another source of fear for those with sensory issues. These persons are more comfortable with an option of a manually flushing commode. Churches can also work on inclusion efforts, making sure special events such as a Christmas program and church camp are welcoming, with the development of modifications as needed. Creating a respite program to give some temporary relief to parents is a caring gesture showing kindness. One church in the Midwest partnered with local nonprofit agencies to create a once a month parent break for any parents in the community who had a child with autism. The child could be dropped off at the church for three hours on a Friday night and the parents could go out and enjoy their evening. The local special needs nonprofit agencies provided qualified childcare and the church paid for the service.

Along with being aware of all the sensory stimuli bombarding the individual and modifying the church environment as needed, places of worship should also consider allowing the autistic person to quietly use an iPad or videos on a phone. Headphones can be offered to prevent the noise from disturbing the other congregants. Many families affected by autism have a desire and a right to worship and feel a part of a spiritual community. Theoretically, churches and places of worship should be the most accepting of environments. Often churches can simply listen to parents about their child or family needs and make simple adjustments for the family such as entering or exiting through a separate door, understanding and being non-judgmental of an odd behavior, or allowing the individual to look at a book during the formal service. Autism friendly churches strive to bring these families into the congregant fold and embrace the opportunity to serve them through identification of needs and a willingness to modify the experience.

Libraries

Public libraries should be places where everyone feels welcomed and inspired. Persons with ASD have traditionally enjoyed libraries for the relatively calm, organized environment. Over time, libraries have become less calm and quiet. The old-fashioned card catalog has been replaced by computerized systems, and the totally silent library of the past has largely been replaced by a noisier environment with beeping scanners and more chatter. Unfortunately, for autistic people and their families, a visit to a busy, noisy public library can be a challenging and regretful experience. However, with a few adjustments, improved staff awareness, and sensitivity to those with autism, libraries can become much more welcoming and present an environment that is autism friendly.

Library staff are renowned for great customer service and a passionate desire to meet the needs of their customers. However, a lack of understanding of the needs of children and adults with autism can unwittingly make customers' experience more difficult and stressful, even painful (Mears, 2017). Many of the unique challenges for libraries serving the neurodiverse population have simple solutions. Autistic people may appreciate organization and like to know how systems work. Libraries can offer tours to the patrons (perhaps some specifically designated for those with ASD) to enable them to understand the layout of the facility and give them a feeling of safety and calm. If maps are available, providing them is also helpful as those with ASD are typically strong visual learners. Signage can serve the same purpose and help the individual with autism feel in control of their experience.

Each library should offer the use of noise-canceling headphones for those with auditory sensitivities. Other calming items that could be available are weighted lap blankets and latex-free gloves. Signage can direct the patrons to available quiet spaces that can be designated for those with special needs. Special sensory friendly story times are usually a popular activity. These programs use props, toys, and tactile objects to offer the listener a variety of ways to process the information being presented. Both the sensory challenged person and the neurotypical population can enjoy the activity that accompanies and enhances the story. For movie activities, a sensory showing of the film would be characterized by softer volume and low lighting. Some libraries offer a special sensory hour when families with a special needs member can visit the library at a quieter, less busy time. Above all, it is important for library staff to understand the basics of autism and be sensitive to the types of behaviors this population might exhibit. Reaching out to families affected by autism and asking them what they need and what would be helpful can be one of the most important steps to becoming autism friendly.

Autism Friendly Workplaces

With the phenomenal increase in the prevalence of autism in the world today, it stands to reason that there will be increasingly more autistic adults entering the workforce. With an estimated 50,000 young people with autism annually reaching the typical working age (Hand, 2020) this topic demands attention. It is estimated that only 35% of adults with ASD are employed, although many could be successful at a job (Shattuck et al, 2012). As with special needs children, many of those adults will require understanding and perhaps simple modifications to become a successful and important team member. Some individuals who participate in an *Autism Friendly Training* may have the responsibility of hiring, training, and retaining employees with certain skills. Others who attend will have a different challenge – working side-by-side with a person who may think differently, and act differently than they do or than what is socially expected.

To create a successful work environment for autistic individuals, both the employer and employees carry a heavy responsibility of a willingness to understand and accept a different perspective. The responsibility to keep autistic workers safe and productive requires a basic understanding of autism. Knowledge is the key for a smooth operation for everyone, and this book and training program offers the necessary knowledge for work-places. This book is not meant to replace or supersede business policies and procedures. Those documents are the first line of operation and employees must familiarize themselves with those procedures and adhere to them for professional and legal reasons.

It is clear that employment opportunities are a major source of concern for young people with ASD and their parents. As children reach adulthood, worries of the future are compounded by the fact that many social services available to children expire once someone reaches adulthood. Young adults are not only eager to earn a living, it is important to families and societies to encourage this new independence. Failure to obtain meaningful employment affects self-confidence of the young adult, who, in many cases, may already suffer from depression and a low sense of self-worth. Promoting and advancing independence makes sense for the worker, the employer, the family, and society in general.

There are many benefits to hiring autistic people. While each person is different, with their own strengths and challenges, people with autism are likely to have some common traits that would be positive attributes for the workplace, such as better than average attendance. Job performance expectations remain consistent with neurotypical employees and companies should value the employee with ASD and not view them as "charity" hire. Companies should hire a person who can perform the duties with reasonable training and support. Some benefits of employing autistic individuals include:

- improved company morale with beneficial neurodiversity exposure and training,
- improved customer perception of the company,
- enriched communication skills of managers and co-workers,
- and increased confidence and comfort level of managers and co-workers in understanding the growing population of people with autism.

The interview process is a critical hurdle in successful employment for a person with ASD. They often have no previous job experience (many times due to unsuccessful interview experiences). As communication skills and social skills are often challenges for the prospective autistic employee, the interview becomes the first challenge and often blockade. Interviewers should be trained to understand the social and communication dynamics of autistic individuals. The company representative should determine whether communication skills are an essential part of the job in question. If not, the interview should be conducted in such a manner so as not to penalize the applicant for poor communication skills. If the job does not require strong social skills, then the employer might consider this fact in the interview process. Some companies might implement an alternative written interview process. The interviewer should look for the applicant's strengths that match a possible assignment. If the interviewer is adept enough to match the applicant's strengths and interest to an available position, this is the first step toward bringing a productive employee onboard. Some companies in the tech industries have an option of an "on-the-job-interview process." Rather than a face-to-face seated interview, they allow the prospective employee to demonstrate their skills.

Once an autistic individual has been successfully hired, the next hurdle is the orientation process. A successful employee orientation for a person with ASD will be clear in setting expectations for the employee and in training them for their position. Employers should give concrete, concise information and avoid general constructs and abstract information. Any visual materials to supplement the auditory message will be helpful. Written materials allow the employee a chance to relate back to the information when needed. Videos for training are also helpful, as those with autism tend to have a visual learning style. A visual list (words or icons) of daily duties or the work plan can be a helpful resource. Employers should present clear, unambiguous information about expected conduct and job performance. There should be a mindfulness to start the process well with a thorough new employee training and ongoing support for identified needs.

Understanding the autistic person and how their autism manifests and displays is critical to acceptance and refraining from harmful stigmatization and judgments. Employers and co-workers may notice a difference in mental organization for the person with autism. These differences may include the following:

- The autistic employee may be very detail oriented.
- They may need instruction on how to begin a task.
- They may not have an idea of how long a task should take.
- They may need help prioritizing.
- They may get upset by too many interruptions.
- They may display "black and white" thinking.

Workplace strategies can often be easily implemented. These accommodations can minimize concerns about communication, sensory issues, social, and organizational skills and include the following:

- consistent schedules and workstations,
- well defined work and conduct expectations (ideally with visual supports),
- a smaller, calm workspace,
- the use of noise-canceling headphones to block office chatter, phones, etc.,
- avoidance of fluorescent lighting – the flicker may not be noticeable to others, but may distress a person with ASD,
- reduction of visual clutter,
- providing a job coach when necessary,
- having a quiet room available if needed for break time,
- and respecting differences in social interaction.

Much of the success of hiring an autistic person depends on matching the employee to the right job. Often jobs that require repetition appeal to persons with ASD. Other employees may hate doing the same task day after day, but the autistic employee may find the repetition comforting. Further, they may be comforted by knowing they have the same seat or workstation each day. Other characteristics of jobs that may appeal to those with autism include:

- regular schedules or routines, sameness,
- a job that reflects their interest and is motivating,
- and a job that has minimal distractions (sound, light, movement, etc.).

Managers, trainers, and co-workers are all important in the successful employment and retention of any worker. Managers and trainers are among the first representatives the new employee encounters as they apply for a job, and co-workers are the all-important people with whom the autistic individual interacts each day. The encounters they have with managers and co-workers often sets the tone for the entire work experience for the autistic person. Professionals should never underestimate the importance of daily interactions with those employees with autism. Whether it is extensive, or a short interaction in passing, the positive and negative interactions have a great impact on the autistic employee.

Vormer (2020) reminds us that we may encounter a boss who has ASD. All of the same suggestions and expectations apply. When communicating with this boss, be direct, clear, and understanding. Do not assume that this manager does not like you if they remain task oriented and minimally social. Be cognizant of the fact that social cues may not be their strong suit when communicating with the staff.

The defining factor of a successful autism friendly program is formation of a cohesive, dedicated team. The goal in a community-based program is to unify the voices of those team members to join into a chorus of hope and encouragement for individuals with autism. The primary component of the *Autism Friendly Training Program* provides needed information which has been created to relate to all the target groups who might serve, work with, or interact with those with ASD. The program also provides highlighted and focused information for first responders, educators, and other groups.

A universal call to action is, "We are all in this together." Educators, civic leaders, retailers, first responders, friends, and family, will all have experiences with autistic individuals. It is important that each community member understand the generalities and the specifics of autism in an effort to harmoniously interact with the growing neurodiverse population. As we are all armed with the necessary knowledge, the citizens of any city can stand shoulder-to-shoulder to support this growing population.

As discussed in Chapter 7, those who wish to solidify their autism friendly knowledge or become an autism friendly presenter would complete one or more of the *Autism Friendly Trainings* which can be found on the AutPlay® Therapy website – www.autplaytherapy.com. The training options include: *Autism Friendly Training, The Autism Friendly Play Therapist* (for mental health professionals), *Autism Friendly Kids*, and *Train the Presenter (Become an Autism Friendly Presenter)*.

9 Becoming an Autism Friendly Presenter

Fuller (2020) stated, "If you have knowledge, let others light their candles in it." Sharing autism friendly knowledge is an amazing gift to give to an individual, an organization, and/or a community. Autism friendly presentations can help teachers, business owners, families, and communities understand the complex and fascinating world of individuals on the autism spectrum. Understanding another's point of view, sensitivities, and communication limitations is essential when navigating the neurodiverse world. Making accommodations and modifications to meet the needs of others can only help societies become better and more inclusive. This chapter highlights the skills, abilities, and processes necessary to become a successful autism friendly presenter. Information will be provided on how autism friendly presenters can increase awareness in their own communities through providing *Autism Friendly Trainings*.

There are a few underlying constructs that guide becoming an autism friendly presenter. One is adhering to unconditional positive regard (A. Vaughan, personal communication, June 13, 2019). Information presented during *Autism Friendly Trainings* is always given in a positive manner. Presenters are asked to never denounce or degrade any other person, idea, or program. While it is sometimes tempting to do so, it is not productive and has no place in an autism friendly presentation. A second construct is professionalism. These presentations are not the place to relive past or current grievances with schools, doctors, law enforcement, the community, etc. It is not a personal forum to talk about controversial topics or promote an opinion. If a question is asked about a controversial topic, the presenter is asked to redirect the audience back to the topic being discussed. Differing ideas, opinions, and beliefs from presentation participants are to be respected but the autism friendly presenter is to remain neutral and stay focused on presenting sound and beneficial information. Presenters should strive to maintain a high degree of professionalism in dress, manner, and information, to maintain the integrity of the program.

A third construct is consistency of information. There are informational guidelines that must be uniformly followed from presenter to presenter to

DOI: 10.4324/9781003105633-10

maintain continuity and integrity in the autism friendly curriculum. An autism friendly presentation being offered in Buffalo, New York should have the same content as one being presented buy a different presenter in Springfield, Missouri. The presentation participants are given an overview of autism and its effect on sensory information, communication, social functioning, and behavior. Emphasis is place on how autism information can empower individuals, businesses, and cities to help improve the life of individuals and families affected by autism. Autism friendly presenters fundamentally adhere to the understanding that those who are aware of the needs of autistic individuals and their families should share their knowledge so that others may learn and share insights. As one small candle can light ten candles and those candles can light a hundred and those can light thousands, one presenter sharing knowledge and understanding of autism can improve the lives of many.

Becoming a Competent Presenter

Presentations are not necessarily easy things to implement – at least not implement well. When we agree to make a presentation, we are really committing ourselves to spending a considerable amount of time preparing and then delivering the presentation in order to share expertise and knowledge. The good news is that it is possible to deliver a meaningful and well executed presentation. A common mistake in presenting is the belief that anyone can present effectively and that being knowledgeable is the same thing as being a good presenter. An individual can have good intentions and be very knowledge in a subject area and yet lack the skills necessary to effectively disseminate their intentions and knowledge to others. Presentation skills can be learned, natural abilities can be harnessed, and those with a desire and passion can become an effective autism friendly presenter.

The commitment to being an effective presenter must be meet with practicalities. No presentation will ever be successful if presenters show up unprepared. Being prepared is making sure that details have been attended to, skills have been fine-tuned, and time has been managed to create a presentation that will allow the presenter to connect with their audience. When delivering a presentation (especially an autism friendly presentation) presenters must be sure that they believe what they are saying. If the belief is not present, the audience will notice, and the presentation will fall apart. Implementing a presentation can take a great deal of preparation but the rewards of effectively communicating to and empowering others is incredibly satisfying.

The University of Southern California (USC) Libraries (2020) highlighted several pragmatic factors to consider which can contribute to delivering an effective presentation:

- *Keep it simple* – The aim is to communicate, not to show off your vocabulary. Using complex words or phrases increases the chance of stumbling over a word and losing your train of thought. Stay to your point and make your point clearly.
- *Emphasize the key points* – Make sure people realize which are the key points of your presentation. Repeat them using different phrasing to help the audience remember them. The goal is for attendees to remember what they need to learn and apply the knowledge outside of the training.
- *Speak loudly enough for everyone in the room to hear you* – Projecting your voice may feel uncomfortably loud at first, but if people cannot hear you, they will not try to listen. However, moderate your voice if you are talking in front of a microphone.
- *Speak slowly and clearly* – Do not rush. Speaking fast makes it harder for people to understand you and signals being nervous.
- *Avoid the use of "fillers"* – Linguists refer to utterances such as um, ah, you know, and like as fillers. They occur most often during transitions from one idea to another and, if expressed too much, are distracting to an audience. The better you know your presentation, the better you can control these verbal tics.
- *Vary your voice quality* – If you always use the same volume and pitch (for example, all loud, or all soft, or in a monotone) during your presentation, your audience will stop listening. Use a higher pitch and volume in your voice when you begin a new point or when emphasizing the transition to a new point.
- *Slow down for key points* – These are also moments in your presentation to consider using body language, such as hand gestures or leaving the podium to point to a slide, to help emphasize key points.
- *Use pauses* – Do not be afraid of short periods of silence. They give you a chance to gather your thoughts, and your audience an opportunity to think about what you have just said.
- *Stand straight and comfortably* – Do not slouch or shuffle about. If you appear bored or uninterested in what you're talking about, the audience will emulate this as well. Wear something comfortable. This is not the time to wear an itchy wool sweater or new shoes for the first time.
- *Hold your head up* – Look around and make eye contact with people in the audience (or at least pretend to). Do not just look at your notes the whole time. Looking up at your audience brings them into the conversation. If you do not include the audience, they will not listen to you.
- *Communicate with body language* – When you are talking to your friends, you naturally use your hands, your facial expression, and your body to add to your communication. Do this in your presentations as well. It will make things far more interesting for the audience.

- *Do not turn your back on the audience and do not fidget* – Neither moving around nor standing still is wrong. Practice both to make yourself comfortable. Even when pointing to a slide, do not turn your back; stand at the side and turn your head towards the audience as you speak.
- *Keep your hands out of your pocket* – This is a natural habit when speaking. One hand in your pocket gives the impression of being relaxed, but both hands in pockets looks too casual and should be avoided.

Some individuals may possess natural abilities in speaking to, communicating, and teaching others. Some individuals may have some skill but need to fine tune their abilities, while others may need to commit extra time to learning how to be an effective presenter. Regardless of the situation, all individuals can improve their presentation skills and adequately administer an *Autism Friendly Training*. Some additional tips to consider for being an effective autism friendly presenter include:

- *Confidence* – To be an interesting and believable presenter, you need to have confidence. The fortunate part is that confidence can be developed over time and will naturally increase the more you present. The *Autism Friendly Training Program* provides presenters with a great deal of material to aid in giving presentations. The knowledge and resources provided will help presenters feel confident.
- *Energy* – Energy is contagious and adds engagement to presentations. Many people will go to see a dynamic and animated speaker because they energize and inspire them. Focus on creating a level of excitement and energy about learning the autism friendly material.
- *Clarity* – Provide clarity to your ideas, opinions, philosophy, and beliefs. Once you are clear and focused, start by communicating your thoughts while continuing to modify and clarify them even more. Be sure that the audience is understanding all the points about being autism friendly. If unsure, ask the participants to make sure they are understanding.
- *Practice* – Practice really does make a person at least closer to perfect. Do not try to memorize all the autism friendly written material. Try to understand the topic to the best of your ability so you can communicate it well during the presentation and meet the time limit. Consider practicing for a friend or a family member and get their feedback on your presentation skills before you offer your first training.
- *Interactivity* – Remember the audience is present with you – involve them. Ask them questions, interact with them, and have them participate – don't just stand in front of them blankly lecturing the whole time.

- *Content Rich* – Your presentation should make several quality points that speak to the audience. They should leave saying "I got a lot of new information I can use." Immerse yourself in the autism friendly materials and continue to learn more about autism than anyone you know. Become an expert and share your insights in your presentations. Teach your audience something they have not heard before.
- *Dress the Part* – How you dress and physically present goes a long way in making a first impression. Be comfortable but dress professionally.
- *PowerPoint/Technology Mastery* – Be familiar and comfortable with any technology you may be using during your presentation. Do not try some form of technology for the first time during a presentation. Also, do not rely on your technology. Remember sometimes technology fails and you should be able to deliver your presentation without any PowerPoint, etc. if you had to (regardless of the content).
- *Organization* – The autism friendly materials come organized for your convenience. Make sure the totality of your presentation day is organized and seamlessly executed. One of the biggest negatives of any presentation is poor organization and thus poor execution.
- *Manage Stress* – It is common to be stressed before a presentation, try picturing yourself impressing the audience. Also, it is important to relax before the presentation. Discover some easy to access relaxation techniques that work for you such as deep breathing, positive thoughts, affirmation cards, or a little bit of light exercise to get the nerves calmed down. Remember, you are there as the expert and you are capable of facilitating the training and giving the audience some very valuable and needed information.
- *Manage your Audience* – It is impossible to fully know what to expect from each audience in a presentation. Presenters will want to be in charge of the presentation and not let a participant take over. Do not let the audience take away needed time with endless questions or personal stories. Also manage and end any discussions that veer into a tangent (off topic) or into arguments or disagreements. Table 9.1 illustrates some common things to do and not do when facilitating an *Autism Friendly Training.*

Table 9.1 Autism Friendly Presentation Dos and Don'ts

Do	Don't
Listen to Participants	Be Judgmental
Provide Empathy	Belittle Opinions
Be Respectful	Ignore Questions
Stay Calm	Claim to Know Everything
Value the Participants	Argue with Participants
Stay Focused on Helping	Criticize Others

- *Enjoy the Process* – It is likely that the topic of autism is something you are passionate about if you are facilitating a presentation. Enjoy the process of speaking to individuals and helping to educate and bring awareness about autism. Remember the good you are doing and the value in what is happening in an autism friendly presentation.

Planning an Autism Friendly Presentation

There is much to consider when presenting an *Autism Friendly Training*. Planning is essential for an effective presentation. Decisions need to be made on the target audience, the location of the event, date, time, and length of the presentation. If possible, finding a co-presenter whose knowledge of autism complements the main speaker adds another dimension to the presentation. A guest motivational speaker is an additional bonus, especially if the presentation is a full or two-day event. The PowerPoint developed by STARS for Autism, available through the AutPlay® Therapy home study/on-line course (www.autplaytherapy.com), assists the presenter in covering the information needed for an *Autism Friendly Training*. Finding an individual, business, or group to sponsor the presentation helps to cover any financial costs. The next steps are determining the setup of the room, writing a schedule for the day, obtaining volunteers, and deciding what materials will be given to each participant.

When creating an *Autism Friendly Training*, the saying "When eating an elephant, take one bite at a time" (Abrams, 2020) nicely applies. The first "bite" of an *Autism Friendly Training* is consideration of the target audience. It may be a group of teachers looking to expand their knowledge to help their students be more successful in the classroom, or school bus drivers looking for ways to help children on the spectrum have a successful start and finish of their school day. Many family members want to have a deeper understanding of their children, grandchildren, niece's, or nephew's behaviors to increase the family's quality of life. An increasing number of business owners are receiving trainings to help better serve autistic individuals as guests and as employees. Restaurants, hair salons and others working in service industry jobs are recognizing the need for increased awareness of those with autism. More and more law enforcement departments, EMTs, firefighters, and paramedics are receiving trainings to help them do their jobs more effectively when interacting with those with ASD. Community leaders interested in helping their cities become autism friendly are increasing in numbers. Some presentations will be a mixture of interested individuals across industries and some might be for a specific group or industry. All presentations will give the basic autism friendly information, but each presentation should be geared for the targeted audience. This is often done by using different examples and illustrations that apply to the specific types of interactions that groups might experience with those with ASD.

The next step is to find a location for the presentation. Many local groups such as firefighters, law enforcement personnel, and businesses have training areas available. Some public libraries have small rooms seating six to eight people up to large auditorium rooms with a capacity of several hundred that can be reserved, often for free. Nonprofit organizations usually have large conference rooms where they allow trainings, especially if the training benefits the population they serve. Public and private schools have areas where a large number of people can be seated. Many settings might offer a room for free in exchange for their particular group attending the training or if a few of their employees or workers can attend the training for free. Don't be afraid to ask a business, nonprofit, or group to provide a space for a training in exchange for a discount on the participation fee or providing some free registrations. Sometimes spaces can be in high demand, so book as early as possible to get the room size needed. The number of people trained per session in an *Autism Friendly Training* is only limited by the size of the room.

The next thing to consider is the date and time of the presentation. Often if the presentation is requested by an organization, the date and time are preset. Businesses may prefer the training completed before regular working hours, while retirees may prefer a lunch presentation at a restaurant. Parents may need evening or weekend programs because of work and childcare considerations. Teachers often prefer a late summer or early fall training as spring is filled with end of the year events. If a particular audience is requesting the training, they will likely have dates and times in mind that work best for them. If you are planning a training for your community, you will want to think about what dates and times might be the most convenient for the most people. Try to avoid holidays and conflicts with any other trainings or large events happening in your community.

The length of the training is the next decision. A brief overview presentation for a luncheon meeting may be 20 minutes. A 90-minute session is the preferred amount of time to adequately cover the material but a lot of information can be given in 45–60 minutes, depending on the needs of the audience. The full autism friendly presentation is usually six hours to have adequate time to talk about the history of autism, communication difficulties, sensory differences, and resulting behaviors. Time is also needed to relate this information to the target audience and allow for a question and answer session at the end of the day. Some trainings will consist of one day to learn about being autism friendly. The second day would be to learn how to be an autism friendly presenter and relating additional information to a specific audience. A full day training is usually 9:00am – 3:00pm (6 solid training hours) as it allows travel time to the venue and a lunch break. It is important to work with businesses and organizations regarding the amount of time they can allocate for a training. If they can only do a one-hour training (something is better than nothing) this is fine, but it is critical to note – the less the training time the less information that can be provided.

Presenters are encouraged to have a co-presenter. A co-presenter shares in the responsibility of preparing and presenting at the training. A co-presenter should have the same basic knowledge as the lead presenter but have different areas of strength. One presenter may have strengths in communication and sensory information, and the other in the history of autism and behavior. Each presenter has their own area of responsibility but can help as needed. A co-presenter is also a safety net in case one of the presenters falls ill or has a family emergency. There are also logistical benefits for having a co-presenter. Managing presentation tasks such as check-in or passing out handouts or supplies is much easier and less time consuming with a co-presenter sharing the duties.

A special guest motivational speaker is always a bright spot at a full day training and is greatly encouraged. Guest speakers usually talk for 20–45 minutes and can be a local or national autism advocate. Guest speakers can have a tremendous impact on the audience by lifting spirits and increasing motivation to continue to work on behalf of those on the autism spectrum. If an in-person speaker is not available, live streaming an autism advocate from another area is also a possibility. A guest speaker can also tape an endorsement of the program to be played at the beginning of the training to help establish credibility. Suggestions for in-person guest speakers are local autism leaders or autistic individuals. Parents, grandparents, teachers, civic leaders, and athletes can be powerful speakers. Anyone who is involved in autism advocacy and respected by the community is a possible guest speaker. The guest speakers add spark, positivity, and a unique perspective to the program. They also allow a break from the enormous amount of information presented. When recruiting a guest speaker, please inform them of the *Autism Friendly Training Program* policy of unconditional positive regard to maintain consistency with the program. Autism friendly presenters will want to complete a small and informal vetting process of the potential guest speaker to learn what they plan to talk about and how they plan to conduct their talk. Guest speakers should be beneficial and helpful by overlapping training content and not create chaos, conflict, promote their own agenda, or be distracting.

Presenters are encouraged to use a multi-sensory approach, such as the Autism Friendly PowerPoint, when giving a presentation. The PowerPoint slides illustrating each of the main categories to be covered, such as introduction, communication, sensory, and behavior are beneficial in keeping the audience's attention. There is no substitute for knowing a plethora of material on the presentation subject that can be easy chosen and shared during presentations. Presenters are encouraged to use the slides as a cue for the material presented. Examples are very powerful and often help the audience remember the concept presented. Presenters are encouraged to practice the presentation aloud several times watching a timer to get "muscle memory" for the amount of material needed for each section. Presenters are encouraged to have written notes, a flashlight, and this book on hand in case of a technology or electrical failure. Some facilities will want a copy of the PowerPoint a few days before the presentation to make sure everything is ready the day of the event. An extra copy of the PowerPoint is always good insurance in case of a problem. Some presenters also email a copy to themselves as further backup. A personal iPad or laptop computer can also save the day in case of technology failure.

As soon as the presentation is ready, a written schedule should be made and agreed upon by all presenters (an example schedule can be found in Appendix 4). No matter what the length of the presentation, three main topics will be covered: communication, sensory, and social behavior. Often there are break-out sessions for those interested in a specific topic, such as developing a disability ministry, creating an autism friendly city, or for those wanting to ask case-specific questions. Break-out sessions can be during lunch to maximize the amount of information presented in a day. Arrangement for sandwiches or pizza should be made earlier and a volunteer assigned to collect money and pick up lunches. For large events, a food truck may be a good idea. Other topics that can be included in a day long presentation include children's autism friendly information, presenter etiquette, service dogs, employment, autism advocacy, local autism resources, and autism resource books. If the presentation is for a specific population, additional information would be given for that population, such as teachers and support staff, police officers, businesses owners and employees, hair stylists, bus drivers, grandparents, or city officials.

Volunteers are a wonderful asset to an autism friendly presentation. Parents, teachers, and other advocates can help set up the room, pass out information, and help break down the room at the end of the event. Try to match the volunteer's skill set with the tasks for the day. Some may enjoy greeting people, others may be technology savvy and can set up the PowerPoint or distance learning. A few volunteers may enjoy the more physical assignments, such as setting up and breaking down the room. Others may be more comfortable making copies and helping before the event. Volunteers will need to be managed by the presenter. They will need to clearly understand their role and duty, when to arrive, and any other specifics that are being asked of them.

A corporate or personal sponsor is helpful with funding training manuals, supplies, and any other expenses for presentations. Banks, insurance offices, and autism advocates will sometimes help financially. Stickers can be placed on the back of materials to indicate appreciation for their support and they can be acknowledged during the training and in print materials as a sponsor or supporter of the training. Often the facility hosting the presentation will help with copies of the agenda and other necessities. Grocery stores, bakeries, and restaurants may also be willing to donate treats for break time. Signage indicating appreciation for the donations lets attendees know who is supporting the presentation. The presenter should reach out to area individuals, businesses, and organizations to acquire financial or other support and lessen the burden for the presenter.

The next step is to advertise the event. Social media is an effective and typically free avenue to let the target audience know about the event. Ask businesses and nonprofit organizations to promote the training on their social media pages and websites. Send media releases to local television and radio stations inviting them to cover the presentation. Presenters should also be willing to appear on local programs to promote the event. Often schools will send home fliers to parents if the content benefits their students. Invite local businesses and agencies who would benefit from an *Autism Friendly Training* to send a representative to the training and ask them to promote the event on their social media platforms. Pre-register participants and send them weekly reminders of the event. Registered participants should be given directions to the venue and availability of parking. A valuable piece of information for all attending is which door to enter for the presentation. A website can be used to register attendees online and send confirmation by email. It is especially important that all registered attendees have an opportunity to request special accommodations as needed, such as a sign language interpreter, extra room for a wheelchair, extra space for a service dog, a food allergy, etc. If the space is limited and becomes full, those wanting to attend are put on a waiting list, so those registered are encouraged to contact the presenters if they need to cancel.

The set-up of the room depends on the size of the room and furniture available. A determination needs to be made before the presentation as to where the speaker will stand, where the attendees will enter, and if there will be a registration table. If there is no registration table, a pass-around sign–in sheet and materials on each chair can speed up the beginning of the presentation and keep things on schedule. If chairs are used, thought should be given to having a center aisle wide enough to support a wheelchair comfortably. Tables are sometimes appropriate for smaller groups. Chairs should be available on one side of the table only, ensuring all participants have a good line of sight to the PowerPoint and presenter. Consideration may be needed for social distancing having only one person per table or two chairs between participants.

The *STARS for Autism Training Manual: Autism Friendly*, by Dr. Linda Barboa and Jan Luck (2017a), is an excellent resource written to correspond with the *Autism Friendly Training* PowerPoint. It reinforces the concepts given in the presentation. It also has a list of terms and acronyms that can be especially useful to the attendees. Presenters are highly encouraged to purchase this resource to aid in the delivery of an *Autism Friendly Training*. The manual is available for purchase through Amazon. com.

The Day of the Presentation

The day of the presentation is full of excitement for both the presenter and the attendees. There can be last-minute details and sometimes a few glitches to address. If the technology person has set up the PowerPoint before the presentation, all presenters and volunteers are healthy, and the electricity stays on, it should be smooth sailing. A volunteer at the door greeting guests as they enter the room makes for a wonderful first impression. Every attendee should be given a schedule for the day. Promotional material such as pencils, pens, notepads and candy provided by a sponsor are always a bonus. Another volunteer checking on last- minute details and technology is an asset. Presenters should mingle with the attendees, welcoming them to the event, and get to know the audience. Masks and hand sanitizer should be available for participants depending on local ordinances and participant needs.

Presenters should remember that unconditional positive regard and respect are primary constructs of autism friendly presentations. As the presentation begins, stay focused on respect for the audience, time, venue, and information being presented. A positive way to start the presentation is, "We respect you and the effort you made to arrive on time. We will be starting now and will stick to the schedule." There may be glitches with technology; that is why a backup outline and resource materials are needed. There may be a full power outage; that is why a flashlight is recommended. If things unexpectedly go off schedule, the presenter should remain calm and work diligently to get things back on track as quickly as possible. General housekeeping information should be shared. Communicate to the attendees the location of restrooms and drinking fountains, ask them to silence any cell phones, and identify the acceptable noise level in hallways if others are in the building. The presenter should be introduced or introduce themselves, giving a short resume of why they are qualified to be presenting the information.

An important topic to talk about before the presentation begins is questions from the audience. Often a well-intended attendee can hijack the presentation and derail the presenter by asking several questions that will be answered in full detail later in the program, or by asking very client-specific questions, causing others to lose interest. A good way to avoid this and stay on schedule is to ask attendees to write down their questions. If they are not answered during the presentation, questions will be given to the presenter to be answered during the designated question and answer time toward the end of the training. If an attendee insists on asking a question, an appropriate response would be "That is a good question. Write it down and I'll answer that during our question and answer session." Be diligent to start every session on time, cover all the identified material, and end the training on time.

Some presenters find it helpful to begin the training with a short icebreaker. This is optional but can sometimes be beneficial to help all involved relax and feel more comfortable as the presentation begins. Some examples icebreakers include:

- *Mirror Moves* – The presenter tells the participants they are going to do a mirroring activity. The presenter will make some moves and the participants must mirror the moves the presenter makes. The presenter can make any type of moves they want (be mindful of those in the audience who might be differently abled) but should try to make it fun. This lasts about one minute. The presenter then asks the participants to find a partner and take turns mirroring each other. This should last around 2–3 minutes.
- *Three Things* – The presenter goes first and shares three things about themselves (the three things can be anything – fun, silly, serious, etc.) The participants are then instructed to find a partner and share with their partner three things about themselves.
- *One Word* – The presenter goes first and describes their current mood in one word. The participants then randomly call out their current mood in one word. You can have people explain their one-word mood descriptor if you want to add more depth to your icebreaker activities, but you can also just go with the flow and enjoy how interesting some of the answers can be.
- *Backwards* – The presenter tells the audience they are going to introduce themselves by saying their name backwards. The presenter goes first by saying their first name but pronouncing it backwards. The presenter then asks the audience (all together) on the count of three to say out loud their name, pronouncing it backward. The presenter then asks the group to do the same thing on the count of three pronouncing the word autism backwards.
- *A Wish for Today* – The presenter begins by sharing a wish for everyone for the training today. This should be something positive like "I wish for you all to feel comfortable and inspired in working with those with ASD." The presenter then asks the participants to randomly call out a wish for the day.

The training should progress along smoothly following the *Autism Friendly Training* materials and guide. Toward the end of the training, the question and answer session should be conducted, making sure to address any questions that where submitted. The wrap-up of the training should include thanking the facility for allowing the presentation, all the presenters for sharing their knowledge, the volunteers for sharing their time, and the sponsors for helping with copies, snacks, etc. Remind the audience to be mindful of unconditional positive regard and respect as they venture into the world of being autism friendly. Be sure to hand out any appropriate certificates or documents and a presentation evaluation (if required). And finally, thank the participants for attending the presentation and for their commitment to serving, working with, and helping those with autism.

The *Autism Friendly Trainings* are available to complete online as a self-paced home study program. The following courses are available on the AutPlay® Therapy website – www.autplaytherapy.com.

- *Autism Friendly Training* – The original training which allows attendees to understand what autism is and how to interact with, serve, and work with those on the autism spectrum. This training promotes awareness of the communication, social, sensory, and behavioral barriers which affect individuals who have autism. Educators, case managers, government employees, medical professionals, first responders, service workers, and professionals across a variety of settings, gain valuable information for working with, serving, and interacting with autistic individuals.
- *Autism Friendly Kids* – Adapted from the original *Autism Friendly Training* but redesigned for elementary aged children. This shorter version is kid friendly, playful, and utilizes the *Albert* book series developed by Jan Luck and Linda Barboa.
- *The Autism Friendly Play Therapist* – Adapted from *Autism Friendly Training*, this training focuses on helping play therapists and other mental health professionals understand what autism is and how to interact with autistic children. This training promotes awareness of the social, sensory, and environmental barriers which affect individuals who have autism. Participants will learn how play is affected and play strengths manifestations common with autistic children. Participants will also learn how to set up an autism friendly play therapy room, how to understand and address behavior in the playroom, and issues to consider when implementing play therapy theories with autistic children.
- *Train the Presenter (Become an Autism Friendly Presenter)* – This training is a train the trainer type training. It is designed for those who would like to become an autism friendly presenter and present these trainings in their own communities and beyond. Participants learn the components of the autism friendly program and how to successfully execute an *Autism Friendly Training*.

This book does not outline specifics for offering the *Autism Friendly Training* via a video format, but this can be an option for presenters. If an in-person event is not possible because of social distancing requirements, location, lack of a venue, difficulty finding childcare, or weather concerns, an on-line group meeting such as Zoom, Google Meet, or a combination of in-person and online presentation may be a viable alternative. Much of the same format would be followed but schedules and other necessary material would be sent to attendees via email. Another possibility is having the live presentation taped to be viewed later. A PowerPoint with voice over can be used to insure consistency in training. Webinar and video training can be just as effective as in person events and can often be more accessible for more people. Presenters will want to make sure they are well versed in organizing and presenting a webinar, as this requires attention to a variety of different issues from an in-person set-up.

10 Autism Friendly City Program

Virtually every community, large or small, in the United States has citizens affected by autism. The population of those diagnosed with ASD continues to grow with the Centers for Disease Control (CDC) (2020) indicating that currently the rate is 1 in 54 individuals will receive an ASD diagnosis. The numbers indicate that cities across the country will have citizens who are on the autism spectrum. Consider the demographics of one such city (St. Louis, Missouri) in the United States. Findings from the Missouri Autism and Developmental Disabilities Monitoring (MOADDM) indicated that 1 in 74 or 1.4% of eight-year-old children in St. Louis and St. Louis City counties were identified with ASD in 2016. 40% of children Identified with ASD received a Comprehensive Developmental Evaluation by age three years. 91% of children identified with ASD had a documented ASD diagnosis. No significant differences in ASD prevalence were found between white and black children but boys were three times more likely to be identified with ASD than girls.

The demographic data from St. Louis parallels the need and prevalence across the United States and serves as a reality that autistic individuals are in every community and these citizens deserve access to community venues and events and full participation in community life. They are present and they are growing in number and communities must adapt to meet their needs. Families living with autism often struggle and feel ostracized socially and are withdrawn in their communities. Many families lose hope and discontinue attempts to take their children to restaurants, retail establishments, playgrounds, churches, and community events. The sad truth is that many affected by autism do not feel welcomed and/or comfortable in their greater community.

An autistic child may lack the developmental processes and sequences a neurotypical child progresses through. It is difficult for the general public to understand autism and the behaviors that tend to accompany the diagnosis. Knowledge is needed for full acceptance and inclusion. When faced with a ASD child displaying overt behavioral aspects (common with autism), the neurotypical person, if uninformed, simply does not know how to react, conceptualize, or progress forward with the child. Is offering help appropriate? Is it better to turn away and let the family handle the

DOI: 10.4324/9781003105633-11

situation? Is it appropriate to ignore? At what point should 911 be called? When there is an understanding of autism and a knowledge of situations that trigger unwanted behaviors, judgements on the correct response are more easily made.

This chapter highlights how a whole city can commit to becoming autism friendly. The course of action and details of completing such a goal are outlined. A city is made up of individuals who work, serve, and learn in a variety of settings and industries. Each of these areas can become a part of a commitment to becoming an autism friendly city. Upon completing an *Autism Friendly Training*, businesses serving the public will be able to welcome a new autism customer base. Families affected by ASD can enter businesses with confidence that they and their differently abled child will be welcomed. They will not need to fear judgements, accusations, and disapproving stares from those who do not understand the complex and challenging neurological disorder of autism.

Citizens of a community must be committed at the city level to be inclusive and free of physical and social barriers to provide equal opportunities to all citizens. Every parent wants this for their family, and every citizen deserves the right of full participation. For this to become a reality, families need support, and the community needs education. But the challenge remaining is to braid the various specific trainings into a strong cable to tie a community together. A city's commitment to becoming autism friendly will be a journey – it will not happen overnight. It will include effort and determination from many individuals. The outcomes of such a project are immeasurable on the quality of life for autistic individuals and the positive inclusion aspects for all the community members.

Establishing a Plan

How does a city begin to take on the task of becoming autism friendly? It often begins with a simple awareness. Gardiner (2018) proposed places that many neurotypical people may take for granted – shops, theatres, cinemas, cafes and restaurants, hairdressers, libraries and museums, public toilets, and public transport – can be particularly challenging environments for autistic people. Unpredictable and unfamiliar noises, lights, smells, crowds, queues, and other events can be overwhelming, and may cause sensory distress – ultimately leading to a meltdown. Meltdowns may present as crying, screaming, kicking, biting, or lashing out. A lack of understanding and awareness of autism among the public can further enhance the distress experienced. Gardiner (2018) established a helpful five-point checklist for cities to create understanding and help families affected by autism.

1. *Customer information* – Providing appropriate visitor and/or customer experience information to help support autistic people and their families.

2. *Staff understanding of autism* – Developing staff training and understanding of autism.
3. *Physical environment* –Making appropriate and reasonable adjustments within the limits of the physical environment to accommodate those with ASD.
4. *Customer experience* – A willingness to be flexible and providing a clear way for autistic people and their families to provide feedback on what is and is not helpful.
5. *Promoting understanding* - Committing to helping increase wider public understanding of autism.

Resnik (2016) proposed that cities should organize by need, interests, and complementary strengths to celebrate diversity that is integrated, multi-level, multiagency and multigenerational, producing richer experiences for everyone and also supporting a life trajectory versus a specific destination, allowing for changes and growth. Several initiatives can be undertaken to begin the process of inclusion for those with ASD. Among the considerations include:

- Involve the broader community, not just the special needs community in addressing pressing issues. Building community support for the continuity of care and important life transitions.
- Coordinate among housing and service agencies at the local, state, and federal levels; promote interagency collaboration, which can increase the efficiency, quality and cost-effectiveness of the housing system and reduce the enormous stress on individuals and their families. Ensure that residential housing for special populations becomes an integral part of a healthy community's housing plan.
- Identify and evaluate what is already working in a community. Build and expand on the community's assets.
- Collaboration is needed to create greater equity, impact, and sustainability for the long-term. Public, private, and charitable interests must be engaged.
- Funding for residential services for aging adults with autism must be expanded to ensure that housing is available regardless of a family's financial situation.
- Cities should consider how the community can work together to restructure the way existing government funding is allocated to housing resources for the developmentally disabled to grow a sustainable real estate supply over time.
- Support the creation of new metrics to track value and quality of life outcomes. Only through collective efforts will public policy advances be made. The best way to change the undesirable statistics for adults with autism is to work together, innovate, demonstrate success, and open more doors for adults looking for jobs, homes, supportive communities, and social network.

Cities do not have to wander aimlessly on their own to go about achieving a more inclusive city. The *Autism Friendly City Training Program* provides city leaders and investors with a blueprint for becoming an autism friendly city. To move forward with autism friendly city planning, the first order of business is to decide what goals the city hopes to achieve. This is an important step in the program development. A decision needs to be made on a goal that is high enough to make a difference in the lives of those affected by autism in the community, yet reasonable enough to be achievable. Successful businesses rely on goal setting to guide them toward yearly and long-term growth. They need a business model and to set goals for the city program.

A realistic goal may be to identify physical and social barriers in the community and to address each of those needs. This is in line with the autism friendly definition presented in this book. This would require offering training to all citizens about autism. The education would be at the level allowing each citizen to become autism friendly. Although not everyone will take advantage of the training, as time goes on, participation may increase. Set a goal to offer free training to every business, church, agency, school, and citizen in general. The objective may include physical analysis of the city parks, city-sponsored activities, and to create plans to improve accessibility for those areas.

As a basic plan of action is formulated, remember that the plan can change as progress is made. It is important to stay flexible and fluid. As time goes by and needs of the community are better identified, the plan may change from the initial outline. Cities should understand from the beginning that although there will be a roadmap in place, bumps and detours may occur. The mindset should be to stay mentally prepared for needed flexibility. A rudimentary plan should include team building, training, marketing and promotion, and community collaboration. An initial process should be established for contacting the citizens of the community. Consider how to get official buy-in from the local elected officials. Think about possible funding sources and who could help pay for materials and training. Set some tentative dates to accomplish the steps of the program.

As the initial guidelines are being considered, network with other communities and cities which are on the same path or who have already completed the *Autism Friendly City Training Program*. Research what has already been done in the immediate area, in the region, in the state. A strong support system for cities may already be in place in another part of the country. Do not be afraid to reach out. Although programs may have fundamental differences, contacts with cities already implementing autism friendly programs may be mutually beneficial sharing ideas and supporting one another.

When the basic plan is formulated, it should be put it in writing. This will become the tool that will be used to present the plan to other stakeholders and to keep the process on track. The following is an example of a plan which can be modified to meet the needs of a community.

1. *Autism Friendly Training* will be offered and customized to each group attending. The following will be invited to free trainings:

   A.   City employees, city officials, autistic adults, and volunteers

       i.   City staff
      ii.   Board of Aldermen (City Council), Mayor
    iii.   Advisory Park Board

         I. When planning playground equipment and park design, include consultations with occupational therapists and architects for full family friendly inclusion parks.
       II. Consult Park Advisory Board regarding city events.
     III. Provide Park Board ear plugs for children and adults sensitive to noise (4th of July celebration, etc.).
     IV. Collaboration may be established with students from local colleges to do service projects with the park system.

   B.   First responders

       i.   Law enforcement
      ii.   Fire fighters
    iii.   EMTs

   C.   Schools and daycares
   D.   Community members
   E.   Family networking and support groups
   F.   Businesses

        i. Restaurants
       ii. Real estate companies
     iii. Insurance companies
     iv. Retail establishments
      v. Salons
     vi. Churches
    vii. Convenience stores
   viii. Banks
     ix. Dentists
      x. Apartment managers & employees
     xi. Entertainment establishments

2. The following training venues may be explored:

   A.   City hall community rooms
   B.   Church rooms

    C.   On site trainings for larger groups, or for retail establishments

    D.   Fire protection district training rooms

    E.   County public safety offices

    F.   Court houses

    G.   University venues

    H.   Public school community spaces

3. The *Autism Friendly Training* to businesses that serve the public, the city employees, and the volunteers may be a one-hour format to introduce the topic and to increase awareness and acceptance. The basic format presented to the businesses and agencies is based on the *Autism Friendly Training Program* described in this book.

4. The training for schools may include all students, administrators, teachers, and auxiliary staff. Staff training may be a more advanced two-hour training based on the *Autism Friendly Training Program, Stars in Her Eyes: Navigating the Maze of Childhood Autism* (Barboa & Obrey, 2017), and *It's NO Biggie: Autism in the Early Childhood Classroom* (Barboa & Datema, 2016).

5. The training to first responders may follow the program *Autism Friendly Training for First Responders* (Barboa & Luck, 2016) and will include the same basic information as other *Autism Friendly Trainings* and include tips on dealing with autistic individuals during emergency situations.

6. The training information and materials in this book are original, copyrighted materials developed for teaching and training the following identified populations. The trainings presented should be supplemented by tangible materials for the attendees to take home for future reference. A complete referenced list can be found in the Resources.

    A.   Adult training materials

        i.   *Autism Friendly Training Manual* (Barboa & Luck, 2017a).

       ii.   *Autism Friendly Training Manual for First Responders* (Barboa & Luck, 2016).

          I.   Supplemental Materials

             a   *Stars in Her Eyes: Navigating the Maze of Childhood Autism* (Barboa & Obrey, 2017) basic Introduction – for all adult trainees.

             b   *Nuts and Bolts of Autism* (Barboa & Luck, 2017b).

    B.   Teaching children about autism is a critical element of this program. The training materials should be chosen according to age and ability.

        i.   *Albert is My Friend: Helping Children Understand Autism* (Luck & Barboa, 2015) for younger children.

    ii. *The Alien Logs of Super Jewels* (Bradshaw, 2014) for older children.

    iii. *Oodles and Skoodles of Friends* (Barboa & Luck, 2018b).

    iv. *Understanding Autism Spectrum Disorder: A Workbook for Children and Teens* (Grant, 2018a) for children and teens.

  C. The Autism Friendly PowerPoint should be used with additional information for the population being trained.

  D. Videos embedded in the slide show will enhance the learning of the audience.

7. Record-keeping and recognition of those completing the program is important.

  A. A participant feedback/evaluation survey may be used.

  B. Day care providers, policemen, EMTs, and others may be obtaining continuing education units or hours.

  C. Certificate of completion given to attendees.

8. Follow up after trainings is a necessary part of the program.

  A. Ongoing postings announcing how the *Autism Friendly Program* is being completed, accomplishments, and progress:

    i. City newsletters

    ii. City social media pages

    iii. Stars for Autism website

    iv. Websites and social media pages of those who received training

    v. Media outlets

  B. Use of training records and future plans for grant applications.

  C. Use of training records and future plans for soliciting donors and contributors.

  D. Entities completing the program may be listed with the global APP Autism Village (autismvillage.com) to help the public locate autism friendly businesses.

  E. Information on sensory friendly sessions showings at local theaters, entertainment centers, bounce houses, bowling alleys, and department stores.

9. Promotions are a positive way to impact the community and distribute information.

  A. Television and radio promotions of the proclamation and events.

  B. State municipal league newsletters.

  C. Newspaper promotions.

  D. Submissions for possible state or national awards.

10. Information dissemination and promotional activity are important parts of the program.

  A. Signage or stickers for business doors.
  B. Media promotions of trained businesses.
  C. Participation with Autism Village (autismvillage.com), creators of the autism village app to help consumers identify autism friendly businesses, churches, organizations, events, etc.
  D. Community baseball games and pep rallies announcing the activities and distributing 911 functional needs assessment forms.
  E. Local fundraisers to assist in the provision of manuals, books, and presentations.

Gathering Support

Like the layers of an onion, the autism friendly city team will require participation at many levels. For logistical reasons, the project will need a person in the leadership role. The leader will be a key person to help mobilize others and keep the project on point. A leadership team will need to be established to assist in the various aspects of the program. The leader and leadership team are integral to the cities success and should be chosen carefully with expectations fully expressed. The responsibility of providing the *Autism Friendly Trainings* will most likely fall to a very special sub-committee of the leadership team. The team will need to make sure that those training the community are capable of doing so – ideally having completed an *Autism Friendly Training*, read this book, and completed a train the presenter training. Both trainings are available for easy access in a home study/online version which can be found on the AutPlay® Therapy website – https://www.autplaytherapy.com/autism-friendly-training/. Time will need to be allocated for all team members to become well-versed in all aspects of autism, as well as being prepared to effectively present an *Autism Friendly Training*.

When conceptualizing and putting together a team, it is crucial to remember that autistic voices can and arguably should be an active part of planning and implementing an autism friendly city. It would be beneficial for those beginning this process to reach out to autistic adults in the community and invite them to be part of the team. For many years decisions about those with autism were made for those with autism without their input. In our present times, there are many autistic adults speaking about the need for individuals on the spectrum to be an active part of any conversation that affects an autistic person. It may not be easy to find someone with ASD to be a part of the team but there should be effort put into this process. At a very minimum, including parents or family members of those with autism on the leadership team will be critical. While neurotypical advocates and professionals in the field can be valuable voices, they are not a substitute for the differently abled sharing their own insights, perspectives, and contributions.

Each member of the leadership team will need to know the division of responsibility. Besides more formal planning meetings, the team may share ideas and progress through Googledocs or similar programs. This is a great way to keep everyone up to date on each aspect of the program. Members of the team will want to meet with the mayor or the city administrator to begin the formal process of the autism friendly city proclamation and to establish a partnership with the city government. The mayor and administrator may request assistance in crafting the official proclamation. They may need written resources to find sample proclamations or may wish to write one specific for the community they serve. The committee may find useful wording by searching past proclamations. Once the proclamation is drafted, the city administrative assistant may be charged with getting it printed, having an official seal attached, and getting suitable frames for the presentation.

The leadership committee will coordinate with the mayor or the administrator to set the official date for the public proclamation. The proclamation will most likely be presented at a regularly scheduled Board of Aldermen meeting. April is acknowledged as Autism Awareness Month; many cities have taken advantage of this highlighted month to present their proclamation. When the date is assigned for the official proclamation, a media blitz begins. Announcements in all factions of social media help inform the community while generating interest and excitement. The event can be promoted daily, and "teaser" memes created leading up to the big event can add to the excitement. On each meme, one goal is announced, along with the date and time of the event. The city may have a magnetic or lighted sign board at City Hall, that can be used to announce the event, and show community pride in becoming autism friendly. Cities will want to highlight all the work they have done and make sure all their community members are aware of this incredibly special designation. It is something the city and the community can feel proud of and no celebration is too small.

The Autism Friendly Proclamation

In the week prior to the meeting, press releases should be sent to all print and broadcast media in the area. The morning of the proclamation, the event can be announced on local TV along with a visual reminder. Personal contact with the local media is important, assuring coverage of the event. Many local news outlets are happy to promote an event such as this. Local families are strongly encouraged to attend, with the assurance the whole family is welcome. Local representatives from area schools, churches, organizations, and businesses are strongly urged to attend the event as are all city, county, and state officials. Even those choosing not to attend will have been alerted of the event and know that it is happening. With the reading of the proclamation and the sounding of the mayor's gavel, the city will officially proclaim itself "Autism Friendly," which gives credibility and cohesiveness to the program.

Many cities hold a small reception when the proclamation is read. Leadership team members will likely be busy behind the scenes enlisting volunteers to help with various aspects of the program, passing out donor sheets to help cover expenses, and outlines of the proposed plan. The team members should be available to answer individual questions, communicate with community members, and provide information to the media. Following the ceremony, thank you notes to all who helped are always appreciated. Initial contacts with those who indicated they would like to become more involved should be made, and another full round of press releases to notify the print and broadcast media that the event had taken place are sent using letterhead stationery or sent as email attachments. A sample press release is provided in Appendix 5 in this book. The informal time at the proclamation event should be used to build relationships with civic leaders who attend and continue to energize community members to stay active and involved as the city moves forward with autism friendly initiatives.

Visiting local school administrators to discuss how the schools can become autism friendly is very important to the community. Schools usually welcome autism awareness and acceptance trainings for teachers and character assemblies for students. The committee should reach out to build a relationship with the local literacy council. Together they can recruit volunteers to read books such as *Albert is My Friend: Helping Children Understand Autism* (Luck & Barboa, 2015) to children and to coordinate opportunities to distribute informational books to children and to teachers or to arrange assemblies to educate children about awareness and acceptance of those with autism.

An online app known as Autism Village (autismvillage.com) posts locations where people around the country have completed the training. Those businesses are publicly registered as autism friendly businesses and organizations. If a family is searching for a certain type of services, they can look on the app to locate autism friendly establishments. For example, a family looking for a pizza in an unfamiliar city can check the app for a pizza restaurant that is autism friendly. The Autism Village app is something that can be shared with business that is often appealing to them. Many businesses will appreciate the chance to be listed in the app and increase their marketing efforts.

The leadership team is encouraged to look for ways to promote the autism friendly designation and to extend a hand to those looking for information about ASD. As April is Autism Awareness Month, the city could consider sponsoring an autism information resource fair. A public venue could be secured, and several providers of autism services could be invited to share their information with the community. This is a good way to get the word out about the city initiative while providing families with needed information about services. This is also an opportunity to meet the city's goals by bringing together local service providers and agencies to network with each other and talk to the public about what they can offer to families.

Addressing First Responders and Service Providers

Team leaders should establish a connection with the Director of County 911 Emergency Communications. They can discuss how the 911 system can best serve people with disabilities and how the team can help facilitate the process. If the county 911 system has a Functional Disabilities Form (example in Appendix 3) registration process, this is a good opportunity for the team to partner with them. This form/registration is something that can be on file indicating there is a person with autism at a residence or associated with a vehicle, etc. The first responders are alerted to this when a call comes in and they can know they will be interacting with an autistic individual. The team can promote the form on social media and make the form available at civic functions. Committee members should go to the local Office of Emergency Management to review public documents showing the emergency plans for the county. The committee can make suggestions that are beneficial to those in the community with disabilities. It is important as the training begins to move forward to also circle back to the 911 manager. The measurable benefit that the project has to the community begins with the very real possibility of saving of lives by the coordination between this city program and the 911 system managers.

Autism Speaks (a national autism organization) completed a study of 1200 parents of children with autism. They found that nearly half (49 percent) of parents reported that a child with autism attempted to wander or run away at least once after age four. Over half of these wandering children (53 percent) went missing long enough to cause worry. A close call with traffic was noted in 65 percent of incidents, and a narrow escape from drowning was reported in 24 percent of the cases. The high probability that a person with autism will require the services of a 911 operator and first responders at some point in their lifetime makes involving and training these professionals an important goal for the leadership team.

The team might assist with designing and printing postcard-sized stickers or magnets for home and auto to alert first responders of an autistic child or adult at a scene. Figure 10.1 provides an example of an identification sticker. The stickers inform the emergency responder that the child may bolt or may not respond to directions. Stickers informing of an adult with autism can also be very helpful. The committee should consider passing them out to first responders and to local families. The 911 dispatchers will learn to identify behaviors that a person with autism might display. The feedback from dispatchers, emergency responders, and a Director of 911 has been very positive,

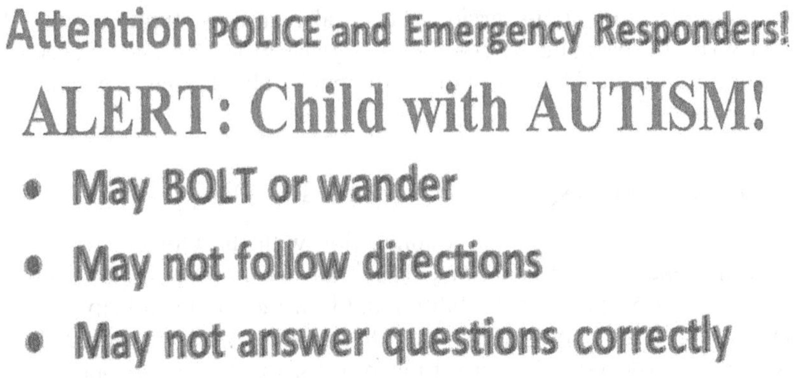

Attention POLICE and Emergency Responders!

ALERT: Child with AUTISM!

- **May BOLT or wander**
- **May not follow directions**
- **May not answer questions correctly**

Figure 10.1 Autism Identification Sticker
Source: Illustration courtesy of STARS for Autism

complete with several success stories of how much the training has helped in various crisis situations. The 911 crew can be an excellent partner in the autism friendly city process.

The training subcommittee of the leadership team can begin to offer the *Autism Friendly Trainings* for law enforcement, fire fighters, EMT professionals, and other first responders several times a year. First responders are a priority group due to the frequency and importance of their interactions with persons with autism. When first responders have a knowledge of working with autistic individuals, it will a make a difference in their approach. Situations involving first responders and those with ASD improve greatly and resolve much more smoothly. If a county/city does not currently have a Functional Disabilities Form registration process, this is a component the leadership team can work on implementing. For those counties/cites who do utilize this process, as people register, in some areas the information goes into a computer base. If a call is made from the residence, the first responders are informed of the special needs at the home. For example, if the person has noise sensitivities, the responders are made aware of this and they may turn off their sirens. If someone in the home has a tendency to bolt and run, the responders will be aware and be cautious with approaching and entering the home. The leadership team can help communicate awareness of the form/registration in the community by passing out informational forms at public events and urging people to register.

Addressing the City/Community Park Board

An outstanding Park Board is an asset to any city. This group of volunteers typically donate long hours to provide events and facilities that enhance the lives of the local citizens. Representatives from the autism friendly leadership team should meet with the area Park Board to discuss ways events and facilities can better meet the needs of the autism community. Some considerations could include assessing areas where modifications could allow those affected by autism to more fully participate and hearing from those in the autism community about issues that may have historically limited participation. A simple suggestion for the Park Board may be to have a quiet room available at city events (such as a 4th of July fireworks celebration) in case an overwhelmed or stressed child or adult needs a retreat from the noise. The room may be equipped with low lighting, weighted blankets, ear plugs, water, and seating for families. A volunteer could be designated as a host in the room, but it is best if parents always remain with the children in the quiet room. Something like this is often an easily implemented service that makes a large difference to the ASD individual.

Working with the Park Board to create a sensory friendly area for the annual Easter egg hunt can be a great benefit to autistic children. A special time set aside with limited crowds is an easy accommodation. If Santa visits City Hall for a pancake breakfast and photos, allow a few minutes early entry for those with sensory needs. If City Hall sponsors a family haunted house for Halloween, a quiet story corner is suggested for those who may need to avoid the chaos. The leadership team can brainstorm ideas with the Park Board throughout the year and have some annual programs established. Playground design and equipment is another area for consideration. The park board, along with members of the team, can gather information and make suggestions for equipment for a more autism friendly park. Landscaping might be used to create a visual barrier, thus discouraging little ones from making a fast exit. More benches for resting areas along the trails may be needed, and other suggestions developed.

There are commercially available recommendations for park equipment designed for those who are differently abled. Often, this equipment is wonderful for all children, not just those with disabilities. An often-commented public favorite is the slide built into the side of a hill. Rather than requiring climbing a ladder, the children can run up a hill, sit on the ground level slide and enjoy the ride down. This would eliminate the problem of children who go part way up the ladder and freeze, unable to go up or down. As children affected by sensory issues often have problems with balance, this design also eliminates the possibility of falling off the ladder. It is a great additional to a park that works well for those children who are differently abled but also very enjoyable for neurotypical children.

Another example of a desirable park feature would be a no-entry water play area where kids can play in the water with no danger of falling in. These look like long troughs that kids can put their hands into, but are safe for children as the troughs are small and the child cannot fall in. Other sensory favorites include chimes and hydrophones, balance beams, and a low ropes course. These are a few examples of ways to redesign the concept of parks to make them more autism friendly yet stay inviting and engaging for neurotypical children and families as well. The ideas provided for first responders and park board staff are simple examples of what might be discussed or implemented. Leadership teams and community members will likely discover many ideas and suggestions that work well for their community. The point is to collaborate and stay open and willing to discover new ways of doing things and recognize the importance of the process.

Conclusion

Building an autism friendly city truly "takes a village." The leadership team will be working hard to make this happen and many other indivi-duals in the community will join the process at different times. Volunteers are invaluable and deserve acknowledgement and praise as many indivi-duals will log many hours of service on the journey of becoming an autism friendly city. As the city moves forward, be assured that the work con-tinues and at one point begins to flow organically. As the first businesses are trained, other businesses will see the value and ask for trainings. As knowledge is shared with teachers and children at the schools, others will see the value and request this information. The team needs to remember that training in schools and some other industries must be an ongoing process with each new year bringing new faculty and students. Fundrais-ing is also a continuous process to help offset current and potential expenses. As trainings increase, the demand for more training manuals requires more funding. Each year more children are diagnosed leading to more grandparents, aunts, uncles, etc. wanting to learn about autism. The need to continue programming will be obvious and necessary.

As a team is formed and a plan created, remember to have the flexibility to shift gears or tweak the plan as needed. There will be times the team needs to reframe a part of the plan and go a different direction. There will be unexpected roadblocks along the way. The team may need to recruit more support for new projects and/or meet routinely with city officials. With the high incidence of autism in the United States, chances are good that someone with some level of influence in the city will have a direct connection to autism and a compassionate heart to help lead the charge in focusing on autism issues. It is normal for the team to start small and allow growth to come naturally. The team should stay diligent and focused on learning and talking to others about the needs of the community. It may take time, but progress will happen. Advocating for the ASD popu-lation is life-changing work. To achieve a status of autism friendly is an exciting adventure for a city. The city needs to celebrate each small accomplishment and success, as those baby steps are the means to ful-filling the autism friendly city goals.

Conclusion

Autism Spectrum Disorder is a worldwide, complex neurodevelopmental disorder that can affect children and adults in all walks of life in multiple ways. A diagnosis can occur in early childhood or into later adulthood. Each treatment plan is as unique as the autistic individual, needing different levels of support in the areas of communication, sensory differences and resulting behaviors. Autism not only affects the individual with the diagnosis, but also affects their immediate and extended families in the many areas of daily life and the greater community in which they navigate. The *Autism Friendly Training Program* offers a basic *Autism Friendly Training* that any individual can compete to increase their own efforts. The *Autism Friendly Training* can be modified to focus on a specific industry such as first responders, hair salons, mental health professionals, dentists, etc. The *Autism Friendly Training* has also been adapted for elementary aged children to learn how to be more autism friendly with their autistic peers.

The *Autism Friendly Training Program* also includes the *Autism Friendly City Training* which offers formal trainings by educated presenters to community leaders, police officers, EMTs, fire fighters, teachers business owners, volunteers and all individuals in the community who want to have a positive effect on the ASD families and others in the community by increasing awareness and acceptance of those on the autism spectrum. The training leads to the proclamation of an *Autism Friendly City* status and guides cities in developing and maintaining this status to better serve their autistic citizens.

Additionally, those who would like to become autism friendly training presenters can complete the *Train the Presenter (Becoming an Autism Friendly Presenter)* training and continue this work by offering trainings in their own communities. Readers will surely discover an *Autism Friendly Training* experience that will meet their needs and situation. This book and additionally offered trainings and materials are designed to continue the original mission of the STARS for Autism organization to provide education and awareness to improve the lives of those with autism.

Now there is a personal call to action. After reading the information in this book, the next step belongs to you. Hopefully you are thinking, "I

DOI: 10.4324/9781003105633-12

have the information, I have the plan, so what do I do next to increase autism awareness and acceptance?" Look around your community. Where do you see a need for an *Autism Friendly Training*? Where can you help those with ASD feel more accepted in the community?

Are you comfortable contacting schools and offering to do an autism in-service for parents, teachers, administrators, support staff, office staff, food service, bus drivers, and custodians? Could you give valuable information to EMTs, police departments, and firefighters? Would you like to give information to business leaders to help businesses better understand their customers and to help autistic employees have a more successful job experience? Do you have the organizational skills to join forces with others and help your community become an *Autism Friendly City*? With the information you have learned in the book, the sky is the limit on what you can do! Go for it, light your candle and make the world a better, brighter place for so many others. Thank you in advance for all that you will do with your knowledge to make the navigation of those affected by autism a smoother more successful journey.

Appendix 1
Terminology and Acronyms

When navigating the maze of autism, there may be some terms and acronyms that are unfamiliar. This guide will give a brief explanation of commonly used terms related to autism and related conditions.

AACs: augmentative and alternative communication devices; electronic devices used to aid in communication for the mostly nonverbal person.

Accommodations: changing one or more things in an environment to make it accessible to an individual with a disability.

Alerting stimulants: things in the environment that make a person more alert or more awake.

Americans with Disabilities Act (ADA): the ADA is a civil rights law that prohibits discrimination against individuals with disabilities in all areas of public life, including jobs, schools, transportation, and all public and private places that are open to the general public.

Anxiety disorders: a diagnosis referring to long lasting anxiety not focused on any one situation.

Applied Behavior Analysis (ABA): a structured behavior-based program for autism implemented by trained professionals.

Aromatherapy: using odors to help individuals. Some smells may be invigorating while others may be soothing.

Articulation: the way a person pronounces their words.

Autism Spectrum Disorder (ASD): a neurodevelopmental disorder which typically affects the areas of the brain in regard to communication and social functioning.

Asperger's syndrome: a form of autism, often characterized by sensory and social challenges.

Aspie: an affectionate term for a person with Asperger's.

Attachment: a person with autism may become highly connected/attached to a random object, person, or toy.

Attention Deficit Hyperactivity Disorder (ADHD): a neurodevelopmental disorder characterized by attention, focus, and hyperactivity struggles.

Auditory sense: the sense of hearing.

Auditory processing: the system by which the brain makes sense of the sounds that are heard.

Auditory sensitivities: when someone may be under or overly sensitive to sounds.

Autism friendly: being aware of social engagement and environmental factors affecting people on the autism spectrum, with modifications to communication methods and physical space to better suit individual's unique and special needs.

Autism Friendly City: a city where citizen have been formally training in autism awareness and acceptance.

Autism Village: an app to help locate autism friendly places and services in a community.

AutPlay ® Therapy: developed by Dr. Robert Jason Grant, an integrative family play therapy approach.

Avoidance behavior: a learned coping mechanism in which the person with autism withdraws from a situation to escape some stimuli that is aversive to them.

Babbling: early speech sounds such as, "mama" or "dada" which are normal speech productions for a baby.

Behavior Intervention Plan (BIP): implemented by a school to address or resolve unwanted behaviors.

Behavioral: any action that is not purely reflexive.

Biomedical: when used about autism it refers to a specific treatment approach that combines the biological considerations of autism when medically treating a person with autism.

Body Language: refers to gestures and facial expressions, communicating with a person's body.

Brushing: a therapy technique used to produce a calming, sensory organizing effect.

Calming skills: persons with autism may need to be taught techniques to calm themselves.

Caregiver: a person who assists or cares for another person, often interchanged with "caretaker."

Casein: a protein in dairy that may have an adverse effect on some people.

ChoicesChat©: short simple chats to have with a child about choices they have made, and what may be a better choice the next time, first identified by Barboa & Obrey in 2015.

Code switching: occurs when a speaker alternates between two or more types of a language.

Co-morbidities/co-occurring: other diagnoses that occur along with the primary issue.

Co-sleeping: sleeping in sensory proximity to another person, where the individual sense the presence of the other person.

Coping skills: coping with unpleasant situations through a variety of adaptive or maladaptive methods.

Cycling: learning a skill, losing the skill, re-learning it, in a cyclical fashion.

Deep pressure: a therapy technique for calming and making sense of incoming sensations.

Depression: a diagnostic condition referring to consistent and detrimental low mood.

Descriptive audio: refers to video that has additional audio content describing aspects of the video that are purely visual and not accessible to blind or visually impaired people.

Desensitization: a treatment that diminishes the responsiveness to a stimulus by repeated exposure.

Developmental milestones: a set of functional skills or age-specific tasks that most children can do by a certain age range.

Diagnostic and Statistical Manual of Mental Disorders (DSM): used as criteria for diagnosing autism and other mental health conditions.

Disclosure: the act of making something known. A person sharing the information that they have a diagnosis.

Discrete Trial Training: an ABA based highly structured method of teaching used by trained professionals.

Distance learning: educating a population that is not physically present at a presentation.

Early intervention: identification and treatment that begins in early childhood.

Echolalia: repetition of a sound, word, or phrase that the child has heard another person say.

Elopement: leaving or wandering away unsupervised.

Emotional support animal: provides emotional comfort to their human.

Executive functioning: the mental process that is used to plan, focus attention, remember instructions, and make decisions successfully.

Expressive language: the language that the person can produce outwardly.

First responders: refers to those in law enforcement and those in emergency medical services.

Flapping: a sensory stimulating activity in which a child flaps their hands or arm.

Fragile X syndrome: refers to a gene mutation that may complicate intellectual development.

Gastrointestinal problems: gastrointestinal discomforts, such as stomach pain, reflux, bowel problems, vomiting or bloating.

Gluten: a protein in some grains that has an adverse effect on some people.

Grief Cycle: the five stages of grief model (or the Kübler-Ross model) postulates that those experiencing grief go through a series of five stages: denial, anger, bargaining, depression, and acceptance.

Gustatory: the sense of taste.

Holistic: focuses on a person's health and well-being and not just their illness or condition.

Homophone: words that sound alike but have different meanings.

Hyperacusis: an abnormal reaction to sound.

Hyperlexia: a splinter skill of being able to decode reading words at a higher level than they can comprehend.

Hypersensitive: abnormally increased sensitivity to sensory input.

Hyposensitive: abnormally decreased sensitivity to sensory input.

Idioms: words with a figurative, non-literal meaning.

Incidental learning: learning that happens informally.

Inclusion: special education services brought into the regular/mainstream classroom to individualize instruction.

Individuals with Disabilities Education Act (IDEA): designed for guaranteeing a free and appropriate public education for all children.

Individual Education Plan/Program (IEP): developed by the parent and the school to provide for the child's educational needs.

Interoception: the sense of the internal state of one's own body.

Interventions: in autism interventions refer to therapies, programs, and treatments designed to help the person with ASD.

Joint attention: communication and a joint focus between two people.

Learned helplessness: providing too much help for a child rather than expecting them to do things for themselves.

Mainstreaming: the process of integrating a child into a typical classroom.

Melatonin: a plant product sold as a supplement.

Meltdowns: overstimulation/dysregulation that results in the child being overwhelmed and losing control.

Modifications: changing expectations to help meet the needs of an individual.

Multi-sensory: using a variety of materials such as visual, auditory, and tactile approaches when presenting material.

Neurodiversity: the range of differences in individual brain function and behavioral traits, often used in relation to autism.

Neurotypical: typical neurological patterns as opposed to neurologically atypical patterns of thought or behavior or autistic thought patterns and behavior.

Obsessive compulsive disorder (OCD): refers to repetitive thoughts and behaviors that are upsetting to the person.

Occupational therapy: a type of therapy that can help balance out sensory challenges.

Olfactory sense: sense of smell.

Parental rights: in the educational system, law designates a parent's rights to information and services.

Perseveration: obsessive repetition of a movement, thought, or sound.

Person first language: emphasizing and recognizing a person before their disability such as "person with autism."

Pervasive Developmental Disorder (PDD): may be used interchangeably with the word "autism" or may refer to a child who has some of the characteristics of ASD.

Pics: desire to eat non-edible objects such as dirt or paper.

Picture Exchange Communication System (PECS®): technique used by specially trained professions, using small pictures to communicate.

Play Therapy: a mental health approach that implements the therapeutic power of play.

Polysemic: multiple meaning words.

Pragmatics: the social aspect of speech, such as greetings and conversational skills.

Predictability: a deep need to know a schedule, transitions, and processes.

PrepChats©: developed by Dr. Linda Barboa as a short preparation chat to help a person prepare for an upcoming event.

Pretend Play: a type of play (typically lacking in children with ASD), which produces pretend, imaginary, and symbolic constructs.

Processing time: the time it takes to process information or input and create a reaction.

Proprioception sense: the sensory system that informs the child of the position of their body in relation to the space around them.

QR codes©: patches registered online, which can be sewn into clothing to be scanned to reveal the child's important identifying information.

Quiet rooms: rooms in a public place such as a theater or church where parents or other adults can calm children who are getting overwhelmed.

Receptive language: the vocabulary that a person can understand (take in) as opposed to what they produce.

Red flags (of autism) early signs of autism that indicate a need for an evaluation or assessment.

Reinforcers: rewards given for behaviors or tasks completed.

Respite: help given by another to take care of the person who has special needs to give the parent or guardian a break.

Rett's Disorder: a genetic disorder that results in behaviors of autism.

Rituals: routines or activities that the person seems compelled to perform, such as flicking a light on and off multiple times.

Scaffolding: the assistance given to a child in learning to complete a task.

Scripting: people repeating segments of conversations or television shows they have heard.

Self-injurious behaviors: behaviors by a person to willfully inflict harm on themselves.

Self-regulation: refers to the ability to self-manage emotions and states.

Self-stimulation: when a person creates stimuli or sensory input for themselves, such as rocking, flapping, or spinning.

Sensory friendly: when accommodations and modifications are made to an environment to address sensory needs of individuals.

Sensory input: the stimulation received through the environment.

Sensory integration: processing information received from the body and the environment.

Sensory overload: when a person is not able to regulate sensory input and is unable to process the information which can lead to a severe reaction.

Sleep/wake phase: the 24-hour pattern of wakefulness and sleep dictated by an internal sleep clock (circadian rhythm).

Social filter: refers to a person's ability to censor their own speech in social situations.

Social skills: skills that are used to communicate with others on a daily basis in a variety of ways including verbal, nonverbal, written, and visual to build relationships.

Social referencing: when a child looks to others for approval or acknowledgement.

Social Stories: developed by Carol Gray, a social story is used to accurately describe a context, skill, achievement, or concept in a specific short story form.

Special needs: usually associated with education and recreation, a term used to signify the need for specialized services or accommodations.

Special Needs Assessment Form: a form filled out by a family which alerts first responders to a person with special needs in the home.

Spectrum disorder: refers to the fact that ASD affects individuals differently and to varying degrees.

Special needs ministry: bringing families into the congregant to serve them through identification and modifications that address their special needs.

Speech therapy: therapy for speech sounds, language development, stuttering, voice, and cognitive problems.

Splinter skills: talents that are far above the rest of the person's abilities.

Stimming: shortened for self-stimulation, or creating sensory input for oneself, such as flapping and spinning, among other things.

Stimuli/stimulus: anything that creates a reaction in the person.

Tactile sense: the sense of touch.

Tactile defensiveness: not wanting to be touched.

Task analysis: breaking down a job into its smaller steps.

Temper tantrum: undesired behavior of a person who wants something or wants to avoid something.

Theory of mind: affects the ability to understand turn-taking, that someone can have a different opinion, and expressions of kindness and comforting to others.

Therapy animal: trained to perform tasks and to do work that eases their handlers' disabilities.

Transitioning: changing from one activity to the next.

Trigger: something that proceeds a reaction or behavior that causes it to happen.

Tuberous sclerosis: a disorder linked to epilepsy and other health impairments.

Unconditional positive regard: a conscience effort to not judge or degrade another person, idea or program.

Vestibular sense: the sense of balance and spatial orientation.

Vestibular activities: jumping, rocking, balancing, swinging, etc.

Visual sense: refers to the sense of sight.

Weighted blanket: a blanket filled with heavy pellets used to reduce anxiety.

Weighted vests: a calming strategy typically used under the direction of an occupational therapist.

Appendix 2

Tips for Being Autism Friendly

1. Do not assume the autistic person has limitations. Half of those diagnosed with ASD have average or above average intelligence.
2. Ask the person how autism affects them.
3. Remember that processing speed and communication might be different from your own.
4. Remember social interactions may look differently, this is not negative; it is different but not a lesser way of doing things.
5. Do not rely on nonverbal messages or body language to communicate a point to someone with autism. Be clear, no passive aggressive behavior.
6. Respect the person's right to decide how they want or do not want to talk about their autism and how they want their autism referenced (person first or identity first).
7. Talk to the autistic person and ask them what they are thinking and feeling; do not assume based on their body language and behavior.
8. Use visual supports (schedules, pictures) when relaying information. Do not communicate only verbally.
9. Do not judge behavior that is different from your own.
10. Look for the strengths the person with autism possesses and try to build upon those strengths.
11. See the world from the person's viewpoint. How are they experiencing what is happening?
12. Do not try to force the person to be like, look like, and act like you. Respect neurodiversity.

Appendix 3

Sample 911 Functional Needs Form

9-1-1 FUNCTIONAL NEEDS INDICATOR REQUEST – IMPORTANT INFORMATION AND INSTRUCTIONS

You are asked to complete this form if you want your police department, fire department, ambulance company or other emergency service agency to know about any functional needs you or your child have when you call 9-1-1 in an emergency. Provided you dial 9-1-1 on a traditional residential phone line, your 9-1-1 call is answered, and the 9-1-1 system automatically displays your address, telephone number, and the name of the person on the phone bill account. (This is not true for wireless or cellular 9-1-1 calls.)

At your request, information can be displayed on the call-taker's screen that will identify the functional needs indicators that have been reported for you, or someone living with you, at your address. These codes will help the call-taker communicate with the caller and provide useful information to the responding public safety agencies.

The information is confidential. It will appear at the call-taker's and dispatcher's screen when a call is entered using the address you provided. This information will be given to the agencies that are responding to help. If you call for an emergency at a location other than the home address that is submitted, the information will not be seen by the call-taker.

The information you provide for input into the 9-1-1 system will need to be verified at least annually. We will either send you a notice or contact you by phone or TTY. It is your responsibility to notify your local County 9-1-1 Emergency Communications Department when there is a change of any information on this form. When filling out the form, please be sure to:

1. Give your telephone number, name, and complete address including any apartment or lot numbers.
2. Check the box(es) that apply.
3. Sign and date the form.

4.   Return the form to the address/email below.

Executive Secretary
Springfield-Greene   County   9-1-1   Emergency   Communications
Department
330 W. Scott Street, Springfield, MO 65802
Questions? Please call #417-829-xxxx or e-mail Executive Secretary
XXXX at XXXX@springfieldmo.gov. Please note: The above phone
number is a NON-emergency number and is only answered during normal
office hours. It should not be used to request police, fire, or EMS response.

Telephone Number _____

Voice [] TTY [] Name of Requestor _____

Name & Age of Person with Functional Needs _____

Address _____

City/Zip Code _____

By submitting this completed form, I am requesting this information be
entered into the database at the Springfield-Greene County 9-1-1 Emergency Communications Department. The information will be used to alert
public safety responders (police, fire, and EMS) that an individual residing
at this address communicates over the phone by a TTY and/or has a disability that may hinder evacuation or transport. This information is confidential and will appear on the call-taker's computer screen when this
address is used. Please check the categories that apply.

[] LSS – Life Support System: Alerts the 9-1-1 call-taker that someone
at this address is linked to equipment required to sustain their life.

[] MI – Mobility Impaired: Alerts the 9-1-1 call-taker that someone at
this address is bedridden, uses a wheelchair or has another mobility
impairment.

[] B – Blind: Alerts the 9-1-1 call-taker that someone at this address is
legally blind.

[] DHH – Deaf or Hard of Hearing: Alerts the 9-1-1 call-taker that
someone at this address is deaf or hard of hearing.

[] TTY – Teletypewriter: Alerts the 9-1-1 call-taker that someone at this
address uses a TTY/TDD to communicate by telephone.

[] SI – Speech Impaired: Alerts the 9-1-1 call-taker that someone at this
address is speech impaired.

[] DD – Developmentally Disabled: Alerts the 9-1-1 call-taker that
someone at this address has some degree of cognitive disability.

[] Other (write here):_____

_____

I understand that I am responsible for notifying Springfield-Greene
County 9-1-1 Emergency Communications Department of any changes to
the above information. I can do this by sending a request to Springfield-

Greene County 9-1-1 ECD, 330 West Scott St., Springfield, MO 65802, by calling 417-829-xxxx, sending a fax to 417-829-xxxx, or emailing the Executive Secretary at xxxx@springfieldmo.gov.

Signed _____ Date _____
Office use only below the line:
Entered Date:_____ By:_____

Appendix 4

Step Guide to Offering an Autism Friendly Presentation

1. Have a desire to actively increase education and awareness about autism spectrum disorder.
2. Read the book: Grant, R. J., Barboa, L., Luck, J., & Obrey, E. (2021). *The Complete Guide to Becoming an Autism Friendly Professional: Working with Individuals, Groups, and Organizations.* Routledge.
3. Complete the basic *Autism Friendly Training.* This training can be completed in person (when the training is offered) or through our online/home study option – www.autplaytherapy.com.
4. Complete the Train the Presenter (Becoming an Autism Friendly Presenter) training. This training can be completed in person (when a training is offered) or through our online/home study option – www.autplaytherapy.com.
5. Decide on the length of your presentation (1 hour, 3 hours, or a full day) and the type of presentation – will it be focused on a specific group or open to everyone in the community?
6. Decide on the cost of the training and a registration process.
7. Choose a date, time, and secure a location for the training.
8. Market and advertise the training.
9. Solicit support from others including volunteers to help with various management issues during the training day.
10. Solicit support from sponsors to help cover any costs associated with the training.
11. Mange registrations for the training and prepare all training materials, supplies, handouts, food, etc. Utilize the materials from the *Autism Friendly Trainings* to help assemble your presentation.
12. Reference chapter seven in this book to make sure you have everything covered for the big day!

Sample Presentation Schedules

Example 1: 20-minute Autism Friendly Presentation for a Service Organization:

5 minutes: What is autism?
5 minutes: Communication and sensory issues
5 minutes: Behavior and social skills difficulties
5 minutes: How can you help in your community?

Example 2: 30-minute Autism Friendly Presentation for a Service Organization:

5 minutes: What is autism?
5 minutes: Communication limitations
5 minutes: Sensory differences
5 minutes: Behaviors
5 minutes: Social navigation
5 minutes: How can you help in your community?

Example 3: 45-minute Autism Friendly presentation:

5 minutes: What is autism?
10 minutes: Communication limitations
10 minutes: Sensory differences
10 minutes: Behaviors
5 minutes: Social navigation
5 minutes: How can you help in your community?

Example 4: 60-minute Autism Friendly Presentation:

10 minutes: What is autism?
10 minutes: Communication limitations
10 minutes: Sensory differences
10 minutes: Behaviors
10 minutes: Social navigation
10 minutes: How can you help in your community?

Example 5: 90-minute Autism Friendly Presentation:

10 minutes: What is autism?
15 minutes: Communication limitations
15 minutes: Sensory differences
10 minutes: *Break*
15 minutes: Behaviors
15 minutes: Social navigation
10 minutes: How can you help in your community?

Example 6: 6-hour Autism Friendly Presentation:

10 minutes: Introductions and Ice Breaker
1 hour: What is autism?
1 hour: Communication limitations
1 hour: Sensory differences
1 hour: *Lunch Break*
1 hour: Behaviors
1 hour: Social navigation
40 minutes: How can you help in your community?

Table A4.1 Sample Autism Friendly Presentation Evaluation

Autism Friendly Training Date, Time Location: Springfield, MO.
Instructor: John Smith Sponsor(s): John Smith Company CE Hours Provided: XXXX

(Please Rate: 1 is poor, 5 is excellent)

Training Objectives	*1*	*2*	*3*	*4*	*5*
Participants will be able to describe autism spectrum disorder and list several characteristics of those who have autism.					
Participants will be able to define the communication, social, behavioral, and sensory issues faced by those with autism.					
Participants will be able to discuss how autistic individuals typically interact and respond in social situations.					
Participants will be able to list several ways to be more effective in communicating and interacting with autistic individuals.					
Overall Evaluation	*1*	*2*	*3*	*4*	*5*
The presenter(s) met my expectations.					
The presenter(s) was knowledgeable about the topic.					
The topic was presented effectively.					
I will be able to use this information in my professional work.					
The facilities were satisfactory.					

If you will be counting this training for CE Hours please indicate your professional and/or professional credentials _____

Additional Comments

Appendix 5
Sample Documents

(Insert STARS or another logo here)

STARS for AUTISM

Autism Friendly Training

This certificate is awarded to:

_____

in recognition of Completion of the Autism Friendly Training.
The participant completed _____ hours of training

on Saturday October 2nd, 2020

Trainer: (trainer name here)

Continuing Education (CE) Information

CE Provider (CE provider name here if applicable)

CE hours and approvals offered (if applicable)

_____

_____

Trainer Signature   Date

Trainer Contact Information

Note: This is a sample certificate. More information is
provided about certificates in the Train the Presenter
(Becoming an Autism Friendly Presenter) training.

Figure A.5.1 Sample Autism Friendly Certificate

<u>PROCLAMATION</u>

WHEREAS autism is a complex disorder that allows our brains to continually collect information about the world around us through our senses such as: vision, hearing, smell, touch, and taste. Which may be over or under the processing of the incoming sensory information that vary throughout a person's lifetime, or even day to do; and

WHEREAS the main challenges associated with autism include communication struggles, sensory issues, difficulty in social interactions, and unusual behaviors; and

WHEREAS while there iscurrently no identified cause or cure for autism, STARS for Autism offers training to virtually every citizen, business, and community to help with public understanding and supporting individuals on the autism spectrum and their families; and

WHEREAS today December 10, 2018, the City of Willard leads the way with the help from STARS for Autism by training City staff, invested Community Business Leaders, and individual citizens in understanding and supporting individuals on the autism spectrum and their families.

   NOW, THEREFORE, I, Corey Hendrickson, Mayor of the City of Willard, Missouri, do hereby proclaim Willard as an

Autism Friendly City

and encourage all citizens to become educated about autism and support non-profit organizations such as STARS for Autism, who bring training to virtually every citizen to help with public understanding and support for individuals on the autism spectrum.

IN WITNESS WHEREOF, I have hereunto set my hand and caused the seal of the City of Willard to be affixed this 10th day of December 2018.

                                        Corey Hendrickson, Mayor

Figure A.5.2 Sample Autism Friendly City Proclamation: (Example 1)

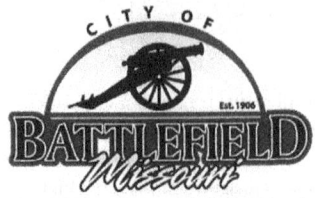

Whereas, Autism is the fastest growing developmental disability in the world today with more than 3.5 million Americans living with autism; and,

Whereas, April has been designated as *World Autism Awareness Month* and President Obama has proclaimed, "The greatness of our Nation lies in the diversity of our people ... Together, we can create a world free of barriers to inclusion and full of understanding and acceptance of the differences that make us strong."; and,

Whereas, Hope lies in an informed public and community committed to providing support and service to individuals diagnosed with autism spectrum disorder and their families; and,

Whereas, The City of Battlefield acknowledges its citizens with autism as valued members of our community and recognizes the importance of education concerning autism; and,

Whereas, Battlefield Missouri, is the home of **Stars for Autism, Inc.,** a not-for-profit organization committed to the mission of educating and training families, professionals, and the general public to better understand this lifelong disorder; and,

Whereas, The City of Battlefield is committed to becoming inclusive and free of physical and social barriers and aspires to provide equal opportunities to all persons with autism; and,

Now, Therefore, Be it Resolved, I Debra Hickey, Mayor of the City of Battlefield, do hereby proclaim on behalf of the Board of Aldermen and the citizens of Battlefield, Missouri, that Battlefield is an autism friendly city; and,

Be It Further Resolved, that the City of Battlefield is dedicated to increasing the awareness and support for individuals with autism, along with education and training for the community.

IN TESTIMONY WHEREOF, I have hereunto set my hand and affixed the seal of the City of Battlefield, this 19th day of April, 2016.

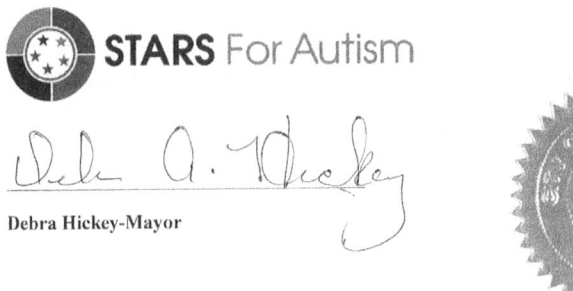

Debra Hickey-Mayor

Figure A.5.3 Sample Autism Friendly City Proclamation: (Example 2)

MAYOR PROCLAIMS BATTLEFIELD
FIRST AUTISM FRIENDLY CITY IN MISSOURI

Mayors across the country are declaring April "Autism Awareness Month". Mayor Debra Hickey of Battlefield, Missouri has taken this a giant step further. The citizens of Battlefield want the world to know that in this city **every day** will be a day of autism awareness. On Tuesday, April 19th, Battlefield City Hall was filled to capacity with an emotional audience as Mayor Hickey made this official proclamation.

Autism is the fastest growing developmental disability in the world today, with more than 3.5 million Americans living with autism. Fueled by an initiative of the non-profit organization *STARS FOR AUTISM*, a new program in Battlefield will offer free training to virtually every citizen to help the public understand and support individuals on the autism spectrum and their families.

The "Autism Friendly Battlefield" project, led by Dr. Linda Barboa, will include collaboration with the city Advisory Park Board to obtain sensory playground equipment and assure that the city activities and programs are autism friendly. The team will offer training to city staff, businesses, emergency responders, churches, and schools in the area in an effort to provide better understanding of autism.

Contact Name: XXX   Contact Number:XXX

Figure A.5.4 Sample Autism Friendly City Press Release

Resources

Autism – What Schools are Missing: Voices for a New Path. 2018 (Barboa & Bradshaw with contribution by Temple Grandin) Amphorae Publishing Group.

With more than half a million children in the United States diagnosed with some degree of autism, public schools are struggling to keep up with the growing needs. The majority of these students are educated in local public schools, and those schools must now step up to the challenge. Schools have both a moral and legal responsibility to educate these children about both academics and social skills. Autism encompasses a very wide spectrum of behaviors and learning problems. The variety of traits they present makes it particularly challenging for teachers and schools to guide these children to adulthood. *Autism – What Schools are Missing: Voices for a New Path* examines the advantages and disadvantages of our public education system for those on the spectrum. This book takes a close look at the strategies and supports that have proven to be successful compared to those that actually increase the educator's burden and limit the student's success. Educators can use the practical strategies detailed in this book to build an enabling environment for this growing population.

Autism Friendly Training Manual: STARS for Autism, Inc. 2017 (Barboa & Luck) KIP Educational Materials.

While it is important to train the population about autism, the availability of competent and knowledgeable trainers is scant. This manual provides an organized, interesting training program, which serves as a practical tool to presenters wanting to train others. Autism: Train the Trainer Manual is designed to accompany each individual attendee's booklet of choice, either *Autism Friendly: STARS for Autism Training Manual* or *Autism Friendly Training for First Responders*. As each participant follows along in his appropriate book, the trainer has at his fingertips this compilation of examples, vignettes, and talking points.

DOI: 10.4324/9781003105633-13

Autism Friendly Training: First Responders. 2016 (Barboa & Luck) KIP Educational Materials.

To become "Autism Friendly" requires learning to identify the factors in our environment and the social issues that affect people living with autism. Becoming "Autism Friendly" allows us to modify our environment, our social behaviors, and our communication to meet each person's individual needs. As autism is the fastest growing developmental disability in the world today, it is imperative for our local heroes to understand the unique needs and challenges of those individuals. This training manual will serve to augment the basic trainings given to First Responders.

Blueprint for an Autism Friendly City: How Battlefield Became the First Autism Friendly City in Missouri. 2016 (Barboa & Luck) KIP Educational Materials.

This book describes the award-winning program which resulted in Battlefield being officially proclaimed the "First Autism Friendly City in Missouri." The reader will become aware of social and environmental factors affecting people on the autism spectrum, and learn to make modifications to meet the special needs of the community.

Autism Presenter's Manual: STARS for Autism. 2019 (Barboa & Luck) KIP Educational Materials.

While it is important to train the population about autism, the availability of competent and knowledgeable presenters is scant. This manual provides an organized, interesting training program, which serves as a practical tool to presenters wanting to train others, or those who just want to obtain a deeper knowledge of autism. *Autism: Presenter's Manual* is designed to accompany each individual attendee's booklet of choice, either *Autism Friendly: STARS for Autism Training Manual* or *Autism Friendly Training for First Responders.* As each participant follows along in his appropriate book, the trainer has at his fingertips this compilation of examples, vignettes, and talking points.

STEPS: Forming a Disability Ministry. 2nd edition. 2018 (Barboa and Allen) Pen it! Publications.

As members of the disability community, many stories and situations tug at our heartstrings. This is never truer than when we hear the pain in the voices of parents as they tell of being rejected in churches because they have a disabled family member. We hear the same scenarios day after day as we listen to parents tell of their failed attempts to attend church. Some are frantically searching for a solution. Others have given up and no longer even try to take the family to church. It is important for families facing the enormous challenge of raising special needs children to find religious support and have the spiritual edification they seek. They want this for themselves, and they need it for their children. STEPS: Forming a

Disability Ministry gives the reader practical solutions for churches large or small wanting to serve these families.

Stars in Her Eyes: Navigating the Maze of Childhood Autism. 2nd edition. 2017 (Barboa & Obrey) Amphorae Publishing Group.

"You have a healthy baby boy!" The words ring like church bells in the ears of new parents. But a child's life does not always follow the road map created in the parents' hearts. Small nagging signs give way to larger, scarier symptoms. Then the dreaded words: "Your child has autism." These words echo in their heads like a freight train blasting through their hopes and dreams. This is a moment that forever defines their family life. Despite the rapidly surging rate of autism, they feel alone. Questions flood their minds. They face an overwhelming search for educational, medical, and social information. *Stars in Her Eyes* is designed to help parents and teachers navigate the dizzying maze of autism. Dr. Barboa shares heartfelt narratives from parents and teachers who have gone before and paved the way. Each contributor gives practical advice from their own unique experiences. Stars in Her Eyes includes powerful yet light-hearted vignettes relating to each topic. The reader will feel that they are sitting in the same room with these authors, enjoying the enlightening conversation of those living with autism on a daily basis.

It's No Biggie: Autism in the Early Childhood Classroom. 2016 (Barboa & Datema) Goldminds Publishing.

It's No Biggie: Autism in the Early Childhood Classroom is designed as an introduction for preschool teachers, childcare workers and others working with young children to best practices in working with all children, but most notably with those on the autism spectrum. The book contains background information on effective early childhood practices, with an emphasis on students who are or may be on the autism spectrum. The very knowledgeable and experienced authors present an overview of autism, specific strategies for the classroom teacher now dealing with those on the autism spectrum, as well as interesting and insightful vignettes that bring these strategies to life. Chapters on the special education process, working with parents and with other professionals, and facing the challenges presented in working with young special needs children provide practical suggestions for both experienced educators, and those new to the world of special education.

Helping Grandparents Understand Autism. 2020 (Barboa & Luck) KIP Educational Materials.

Grandparents, here is the book you have been looking for! *Helping Grandparents Understand Autism* is a Grandparent Friendly Guide by Dr. Linda Barboa and Jan Luck. It was written to help you understand this complex disorder and how it affects your grandchild. It tells how communication difficulties and sensory issues may affect your grandchild's behavior. It explains many of the challenges that children with autism face. Best of all it helps you understand your grandchild and gives you practical ways to help them be more successful in family life. Strategies are provided to strengthen your relationship with the child. Thank you for helping your grandchild!

Restaurant Autism Friendly Training. 2018 (Barboa & Luck) KIP Educational Materials.

As a nation, Americans eat out between four and five times a week. It is a common convenience that most families take for granted. For families with a child with autism spectrum disorder (ASD), that ease and convenience is often replaced with embarrassment and rejection. The family who planned a celebration may feel that they were subjected instead to a nightmare experience. The communication challenges they face, complicated by common characteristics of people with autism, can combine to create an unhappy experience for the family, the restaurant staff, and the other patrons. Enlightened restaurants are beginning to realize that the ensuing meltdowns can be prevented rather than handling them when they are full-blown. With some small changes, staff understanding, and tweaking of routine procedures, many problems and melt-downs can be prevented. With smooth family service, the family has the quality dining experience and the restaurant has retained a happy customer, more likely to return to patronize that establishment again.

Bus Driver Autism Friendly Training Manual. 2017 (Barboa & Luck) KIP Educational Materials.

The importance of the interaction that the school support staff have with students is often overlooked. Bus drivers play a critical role in preparing the student for the day. They also set the tone for a happy family evening. In the *Bus Driver Autism Friendly Training Manual,* the authors give readers a no-nonsense informative account of what bus drivers and attendants need to know to meet these expectations. The design of the book lends itself to be used as an in-service for the transportation staff.

Beautician Autism Friendly Training. 2018 (Barboa & Luck) KIP Educational Materials.

Autism is a complex disorder. As we go through our everyday lives, our brains continually collect information about the world around us through our senses. In autism, the senses may be over or under processing the incoming stimuli. People with autism are not able to make sense of the incoming sensory information. As a beautician, your challenge is two-fold: to meet the client's grooming needs and to do that in a non-traumatizing way. With 3.5 million Americans identified as being on the autism spectrum there is a good chance that all beauticians and barbers will serve clients with these characteristics. Whether you are a professional cosmetologist or a parent who has decided to take on this task at home with your own children, the practical suggestions in this book should prove helpful.

Teachers Autism Friendly Training. 2018 (Barboa & Luck) KIP Educational Materials.

Autism is the fastest growing developmental disability in the world today. Teachers need practical suggestions to create classrooms free of physical and social barriers to student success. This training manual is designed to be used with *Autism Friendly Training* to address those needs. Awareness and understanding of autism have improved markedly in recent times. However, there is still a long way to go. Misconceptions are rampant and damaging. Knowledge is power, and this program provides practical strategies to assist teachers in their quest for improved student outcomes.

Autism Friendly Workplace: A Guide for Employers and Co-Workers. 2018 (Barboa & Luck) KIP Educational Materials.

With the phenomenal increase in the prevalence of autism in the world today, there will be increasingly more adults on the autism spectrum entering the workforce. With an estimated 50,000 young people with autism reaching the typical working age each year, this topic demands attention. The employment rate is low among adults with autism, although many are high functioning. Many of those adults will require understanding and perhaps simple modifications to become successful and important team members. Employers and co-workers may have the responsibility of hiring, training, and retaining employees with certain skills. Others will have a different challenge working side by side with a person who may think differently and act differently than they do. To have a successful work environment, both of those roles carry a heavy responsibility, understanding of a different perspective, and a loving spirit. The responsibility to keep this group of workers safe and productive requires a basic understanding of autism. Knowledge is power, and in this book, we offer you that knowledge.

The Nuts and Bolts of Autism: Just the Facts! 2016 (Luck & Barboa) KIP Educational Materials

The Nuts and Bolts of Autism: Just the Facts! is a quick, easy to read booklet designed to answer some of the most frequently asked questions about autism. The authors use a no-frills approach to provide information in the most concise and convenient format. Written for readers seeking the basic facts, this book is a good place to start. Extended family members and community members, along with retail and service providers, will get a valuable introduction to autism.

Tic Toc Autism Clock: A Guide to Your 24/7 Plan. Second edition 2015 (Obrey & Luck) Pen it! Publications.

Autism does not sleep. When night falls, families everywhere tuck their children into bed for what will typically be a good night's sleep, but the care required by the child with special needs continues around the clock. Like grandfather's pocket watch, if not wound consistently, the ticking will stop. Without proper early intervention there is a very real danger of watching a child fade from this world into a world he has created in his own mind. There is a push toward early diagnosis and education because it is universally understood that early intervention is vital for optimal gain. The younger a child is, the better chance of increased efficacy and possible re-growth of neural pathways. Teachers and therapists often provide some services during the day, but the family is the 24/7 team.

Taking it to the Streets: How to be an Advocate. 2019 (Barboa and Obrey) KIP Educational Materials.

There are many directions a caring individual can take to advocate for others. Getting involved can be accomplished in a number of fun and interesting ways. Advocacy includes speaking, writing, or acting on behalf of an interest. In this manual we will examine how the reader can become active in those avenues. For the reader who is already an active advocate, this book suggests ways to take advocacy to the next level.

AutPlay® Therapy Play and Social Skills Groups: A Ten Session Model. 2020 (Grant & Turner-Bumberry) Routledge.

This book provides practitioners with a step-by-step guide for implementing a social skills group to help autistic children and adolescents improve on their play and social navigation needs in a fun and engaging way. This unique 10-session group model incorporates the AutPlay Therapy approach focused on relational and play methods. Group setup, protocol, and structured play therapy interventions are presented and explained for easy implementation by professionals. Also included are parent implemented interventions that allow parents and/or caregivers to become co-change agents in the group process and learn how to successfully implement AutPlay groups. Any practitioner or professional who works with children and adolescents with autism spectrum disorder will find this resource to be a unique and valuable guide to effectively implementing social skills groups.

AutPlay® Therapy for Children and Adolescents on the Autism Spectrum: A Behavioral Play-Based Approach. Third edition 2017 (Grant) Routledge.

AutPlay Therapy is an integrative family play therapy approach to help address the mental health needs of autistic children and adolescents and other neurodivergent children. This innovative new model contains a parent-training component (wherein parents are co-change agents and implement directive play therapy interventions in the home setting) and can be utilized in any setting where children and adolescents with an autism disorder, ADHD, dysregulation issues, or other neurodevelopmental disorders are treated. This comprehensive resource outlines the AutPlay Therapy process and offers a breakdown of therapy phases along with numerous assessment materials and over 30 directive play therapy techniques.

Play-Based Interventions for Autism Spectrum Disorder and Other Developmental Disabilities. 2017 (Grant) Routledge.

This book contains a wide selection of play therapy interventions for use with autistic children and adolescents, dysregulation issues, or other developmental disabilities. The structured interventions focus on improvement in social navigation, emotional regulation, connection and relationship development, and anxiety reduction. Special considerations for implementing structured interventions and an intervention tracking sheet are also presented. This valuable tool is a must have for both professionals and parents working on skill development with these populations.

Understanding Sensory Processing Challenges: A Workbook for Children and Teens. 2018 (Grant) AutPlay® Publishing.

Children and teens who experience sensory challenges often find it difficult to understand the issues they are struggling with and why they are struggling with these issues. *Understanding Sensory Processing Challenges: A Workbook for Children and Teens* is designed for professionals and parents to work with children who are experiencing sensory processioning struggles. The workbook offers worksheets, play therapy interventions, and resources specifically designed to address sensory challenges. Each worksheet covers a different topic related to gaining awareness about sensory challenges and helping children and teens better understand what it means to have sensory struggles. Through each worksheet, children and teens have the opportunity to express their thoughts and feelings and ask questions. The workbook also provides a guide for professionals and parents offering instructions, information, and suggestions for implementing and processing through each worksheet page. Several play therapy interventions targeting improvement in sensory integration are described for easy implementation by both professionals and parents. The concept of a sensory play diet is fully explored equipping those who work with children and teens with sensory challenges to effectively implement sensory play activities to improve sensory issues. Professionals and parents will find *Understanding Sensory Processing Challenges* a valuable tool they will use again and again in working with children and teens with sensory issues. Children and teens will enjoy the engaging worksheets as they discover and process through their complex diagnosis.

Understanding Autism Spectrum Disorder: A Workbook for Children and Teens. 2018 (Grant) AutPlay® Publishing.

Children and teens often have a challenging time understanding their autism spectrum disorder diagnosis. This workbook is designed to help professionals and parents explain autism to children and teens. Each worksheet covers a different topic related to gaining awareness about autism and helping children and teens better understand what it means to have an autism spectrum disorder. Through each worksheet, children and teens have the opportunity to express their thoughts and feelings and ask questions. The workbook also provides a guide for professionals and parents offering instructions, information, and suggestions for implementing and processing through each worksheet page. Professionals and parents will find *Understanding Autism Spectrum Disorder* a valuable tool in working with children and teens with autism. Children and teens will enjoy the engaging worksheets as they discover and process through their complex diagnosis.

Children's Books

Albert is My Friend: Helping Children Understand Autism. Second edition 2017 (Luck & Barboa) Goldminds Publishing. Also in Spanish, Dutch, and German.

Meet Albert. He doesn't say much, but has a lot of great ideas. Mary Louise likes Albert even though he is different from her other friends. Albert and Mary Louise want everyone to know that being different is okay. *Albert is My Friend: Helping Children to Understand Autism* is about the friendship between a young boy, Albert, who is on the autism spectrum and his friend, Mary Louise. Together they describe and explain some common autism behaviors at a child's level of understanding. This read-aloud book has engaging color pictures that will hold the attention of children and adults. This book presents a positive attitude and is a must read for family members, teachers, and community members.

Albert Thinks About His Future: Helping Children Understand Autism. 2017 (Luck & Barboa) Goldminds Publishing.

Albert Thinks About His Future is the engaging story of Albert, a young preverbal boy on the autism spectrum, as he thinks about the many possibilities he has for his future. His family and friends encourage him to think about his strengths and interests as he considers his potential occupations.

Albert Goes to Camp: Helping Children Understand Autism. 2015 (Luck & Barboa) KIP Educational Materials.

Albert Goes to Camp; Helping Children Understand Autism is one in a series of books designed to help children understand autism. This book follows Albert, a young boy on the autism spectrum through his experience at camp. Albert's experiences will help prepare a young reader for his own upcoming trip to camp. This read-aloud book has engaging color pictures that will charm children and adults alike. Albert presents a positive attitude and is a must read for families and schools.

Albert Goes to Church: Helping Children Understand Autism. 2015 (Barboa & Luck) KIP Educational Materials.

As part of the "Albert is My Friend" series, this book continues to help children learn about autism. In Albert Goes to Church, the reader follows Albert through the experience of going to church. The reader comes to understand how the sensory experience of attending church can affect a child. This book is presented in a positive mindset. The colorful pictures make this book perfect as a read-aloud book.

Albert Goes to School: Helping Teachers and Children Understand Autism. 2015 (Barboa & Luck) KIP Educational Materials.

Albert Goes to School: Helping Teachers and Children Understand Autism describes the challenges that Albert faces at school, as a child with autism. As the readers follow Albert through his school day, they gain insight into his behaviors. This read-aloud book is colorfully designed to hold the attention of both children and adults. This book gives the reader a glimpse into Albert's world. *Albert Goes to School* presents a positive attitude and is a must-read for children, family members, teachers and community members.

Albert Builds a Friendship: Helping Children Understand Autism. 2018 (Barboa & Luck). Goldminds Publishing.

Albert is listening carefully as his teacher, Miss Dixie, talks about friendship. Albert knows he has friends, but he does not have a ship! The beautiful illustrations help children understand about friendship and, like Albert, realize that they each have a "Friend Ship" in their heart.

Oodles and Skoodles of Friends. 2018 (Luck & Barboa) Goldminds Publishing.

Oodles and Skoodles of Friends is a remarkable book for children pre-school to 2nd grade. It is filled with delightful illustrations. The energetic alliteration and rhyme capture the imagination and hold the attention of young children. There is an underlying theme of friendship and acceptance as children learn number concepts by counting a variety of friends.

Lost Dog Doodles: A Raspberry Kid's Adventure. 2018 (Barboa & Luck) Pen it! Publications.

Sophie Sigour's dog, Doodles, has disappeared. She calls on her friends in the Raspberry Noodles Gang to help. Can they find her beloved Doodles and bring him back home to her? They have a plan. . . they can . . . they can.

Learning Manners with the Raspberry Noodles Kids. 2019 (Barboa & Luck) Pen it! Publications.

Learning Manners is a must have book for children, preschool to 2nd grade. The fourth book in the Raspberry Noodles Kids series continues the tradition of imaginative rhyme, alliteration and illustrations to reinforce manners in a positive fun way. Children will learn the appropriate times to say "please" and "thank you", turn taking, swallowing food before you talk, and many more important skills from their Raspberry Noodles friends.

Scared of Santa: A Raspberry Noodle Adventure. 2017 (Luck & Barboa) Goldminds Publishing.

Scared of Santa is the second book in the Raspberry Noodles Kids series. It continues the tradition of energetic alliteration and rhyme with delightful illustrations. Friendship and acceptance are demonstrated as Tanicus True's friends find ways to help him visit Santa. Children of all ages will enjoy this story of true Christmas joy.

Service Dog Dingo. 2019 (Barboa & Luck) Pen it! Publications. Also available in French.

Dingo was a lonely little dog on the streets until trainer Shawn took him in and trained him to be a Service Dog. Now Dingo is happy to be of service to his owner, Tilly.

Friends of Many Shapes and Colors. 2020 (Barboa and Pfennig) KIP Educational Materials.

All the colorful shapes were wonderful friends. They played games together in the spring, summer, winter and fall. One day the shapes noticed that they were all different and started teasing each other. This made all the shapes sad and lonely. Then the shapes agreed that they did not need to look alike to be friends. This book carries an anti-bullying message as it teaches children about diversity. The colorful, playful images will delight the young children as they learn about shapes. This book is a must for every classroom of young children, and every household.

References

Abrams, C. (2020). *Brainy Quote.* https://www.brainyquote.com/quotes/creighton_a brams_207381

Allen, J. (2019, August 8). A guide to visiting theme parks with a child on the autism spectrum. *The Points Guy.* https://thepointsguy.com/guide/visiting-theme-parks-child-on-autism-spectrum/

American Psychiatric Association. (2014). *Diagnostic and statistical manual of mental disorders (5ᵗʰ ed.).* American Psychiatric Association.

Attwood, T., & Garnett, M. (2013). *CBT to help young people with Asperger's syndrome (autism spectrum disorder) to understand and express affection.* Jessica Kingsley Publishers.

Autism Action Partnership. (2020). Frequently asked questions. https://autismaction.org/aboutautism/faqs/

Autism Society of America. (2020). What is autism?https://www.autism-society.org/what-is/

Autism Speaks. (2020). What is autism?https://www.autismspeaks.org/what-autism

Barboa, L. & Allen, S. (2018). *STEPS: Forming a disability ministry.* Pen it! Publications.

Barboa, L. & Bradshaw, B. (2018). *Autism – what schools are missing: Voices for a new path.* Goldminds Publishing.

Barboa, L. & Datema, M. (2016). *It's no biggie: Autism in the early childhood classroom.* Goldminds Publishing.

Barboa, L., & Luck, J. (2016) *Autism friendly training for first responders.* KIP Educational Materials.

Barboa, L. & Luck, J. (2017a). *Autism friendly training manual.* KIP Educational Materials.

Barboa, L., & Luck. (2017b). *Nuts and bolts of autism.* KIP Educational Materials.

Barboa, L. & Luck, J. (2018a). *Restaurant autism friendly training manual.* KIP Educational Materials.

Barboa, L., & Luck, J. (2018b). *Oodles and skoodles of friends.* Goldminds Publishing.

Barboa, L. & Obrey, E. (2017). *Stars in her eyes: Navigating the maze of childhood autism.* Goldminds Publishing.

Baron-Cohen, S. (2019, April 30). The concept of neurodiversity is dividing the autism community. *Scientific American.* https://blogs.scientificamerican.com/observations/the-concept-of-neurodiversity-is-dividing-the-autism-community/

Becker, J. (2020). 17 staggering statistics about our shopping habits. *Becomingminimalist.* https://www.becomingminimalist.com/shopping-statistics/

Bennie, M. (2016, April 12). What is neurodiversity?Autism Awareness Centre. https://autismawarenesscentre.com/un-adopts-new-goals-disabilities/

Bill Vicars. (2017, November 7). Learn sign language: Lesson 01 [Video]. YouTube. https://www.youtube.com/watch?v=DaMjr4AfYA0&feature=emb_logo

Bonis, S. (2016). Stress and parents of children with autism: A review of literature. *Issues in Mental Health Nursing*, 37 (3), 153–163. doi:10.3109/01612840.2015.1116030

Botha, M., & Frost, D. M. (2019). Extending the minority stress model to understand mental health problems experienced by the autistic population. *Society and Mental Health*. doi:10.1177/2156869318804297

Bradshaw, B. (2014). *The alien logs of super jewels*. Goldminds Publishing.

Carr, S. (2017, September 22). The tricky path to employment is trickier when you're autistic: Autistic children grow up to be autistic adults. Our society doesn't give them the support they need. *Slate*. https://slate.com/business/2017/09/how-autism-complicates-the-path-to-employment.html

Centers for Disease Control and Prevention (CDC). (2020). Autism spectrum disorder. https://www.cdc.gov/ncbddd/autism/index.html

Chasen, L. R. (2014). *Engaging mirror neurons inspire connection and social emotional development in children and teens on the autism spectrum*. Jessica Kingsley Publishers.

Children's Hospital Los Angeles. (2014, December 15). Culture factors influence how we experience autism. https://www.chla.org/blog/behavior-and-development/culture-factors-influence-how-we-experience-autism

Coplan, J. (2010). *Making sense of autistic spectrum disorders*. Bantam Books.

D'Amico, M., & Lalonde, C. (2017). The effectiveness of art therapy for teaching social skills to children with autism spectrum disorder. *Art Therapy: Journal of the American Art Therapy Association*, 34 (4), 176–182.

Enoch, J., McDonald, L., Jones, L. (2019). Evaluating whether sight is the most valued sense. *JAMA Ophthalmology*, 137, 11.

Exkorn, K.S. (2005). *The autism sourcebook*. HarperCollins Publishers.

Fuller, M. (2020). *Brainy Quote*. https://www.brainyquote.com/quotes/margaret_fuller_131958?utm_source=ios&utm_medium=app&utm_campaign=131958

Galanopoulous, A., Robertson, D., Spain, D., & Murphy, C. (2014). Mental health supplement. *Your Autism Magazine*, 8 (4), Winter.

Gardiner, D. (2018). Autism-friendly cities: Making a world of difference. *The Knowledge Exchange*. https://theknowledgeexchangeblog.com/2018/11/26/autism-friendly-cities-making-a-world-of-difference/

Gates, G. (2019). *Trauma, stigma, and autism: Developing resilience and loosening the grip of shame*. Jessica Kingsley.

Gerhardt, P. (2004). Food for thought: Adulthood. In C. Sicile-Kira (Ed.). *Autism spectrum disorders: The complete guide to understanding autism, Asperger's syndrome, pervasive developmental disorder, and other ASDs*. Berkley Publishing Group.

Golnik A., Ireland, M. & Borowsky, T. (2009). Medical Homes for Children with Autism. *Official Journal of the American Academy of Pediatrics*, 123, 966–971 doi:10.1542/peds.2008 1321

Grandin, T. (2012). *Different not less: Inspiring stories of achievement and successful employment from adults with autism, Asperger's, and ADHD*. Future Horizons.

Grant, R. J. (2015). Family play counseling with children affected by autism. In E. J. Green, J. N. Baggerly, A. C. Myrick (Eds.), *Counseling families: Play based treatments* (pp. 109–125). Rowman & Littlefield.

Grant, R. J. (2017a). *Autplay therapy for children and adolescents on the autism spectrum.* (3rd ed.). Routledge.

Grant, R. J. (2017b). *Play based interventions for autism spectrum disorder and other developmental disabilities.* Routledge.

Grant, R. J. (2018a). *Understanding autism spectrum disorder: A workbook for children and teens.* AutPlay Publishing.

Grant, R. J. (2018b). *Understanding sensory processing challenges: A workbook for children and teens.* AutPlay Publishing.

Grant, R. J. (2020). Play therapy and the autism parent. *Play Therapy,* 15 (2).

Grant, R. J., & Turner-Bumberry, T. (2020). *AutPlay therapy play and social skill groups: A ten session model.* Routledge.

Grant, R. J. (in press). Foreword. In E.Gil, & A. A. Drewes (Eds.), *Cultural Issues in Play Therapy* (2nd ed.). Guilford Press.

Grant, R. J., Stone, J., & Mellenthin, C. (2020). *Play therapy theories and perspectives: A collection of thoughts in the field.* Routledge.

Gray, C. (2020). https://carolgraysocialstories.com/.

Gregory, C. (2020, September 23). The five stages of grief, an examination of the Kübler-Ross Model. *PSYCOM.* https://www.psycom.net/depression.central.grief.html

Hamm, T. (2020). Don't eat out as often. *The Simple Dollar.* https://www.thesimpledollar.com/save-money/dont-eat-out-as-often/

Hand, B. (2020). Meet Dr. Brittany Hand. *Autism Speaks.* https://www.autismspeaks.org/profile/meet-dr-brittany-hand

Hendricks, D. (2010). Employment and adults with autism spectrum disorders: Challenges and strategies for success. *Journal of Vocational Rehabilitation,* 32 (2), 125–134 doi:10.3233/JVR-2010-0502

Hoover, D. W. (2015). The effects of psychological trauma on children with autism spectrum disorders: A research review. *Journal of Autism and Developmental Disorders,* 2 (3), 287–299.

Howard, A. R., Copeland, R., Lindaman, S., & Cross, R. (2017). Theraplay impact on parents and children with autism spectrum disorder: improvements in affect, joint attention, and social cooperation. *International Journal of Play Therapy,* 27, 56–68.

International Board of Credentialing and Continuing Education Standards (IBCCES). (2020). Autism friendly isn't good enough. https://ibcces.org/cac-info/

Kasari, C., Dean, M., Kretzmann, M., Shih, W., Orlich, F., Whitney, R., Landa, R., Lord, C., & King, B. (2016). Children with autism spectrum disorder and social skills groups at school: a randomized trial comparing intervention approach and peer composition. *Journal of Child Psychology and Psychiatry,* 57 (2), 171–179.

Kingsley, E. (1987). Welcome to Holland. National Down Syndrome Society. https://www.ndss.org/lifespan/a-parents-perspective/

Koenig, K. (2012). *Practical social skills for autism spectrum disorders.* W. W. Norton.

Luck, J., & Barboa, B. (2015). *Albert is my friend: Helping children understand autism.* (2nd ed.). Goldminds Publishing.

Lutz, A. (2020, June 23). When autism advocacy is "partial." *Psychology Today.* https://www.psychologytoday.com/us/blog/inspectrum/202006/when-autism-advocacy-is-partial

Marshall, K. (2019, October 1). A small village becomes an autism supportive community. *Autism Spectrum News.* https://autismspectrumnews.org/a-small-village-becomes-an-autism-supportive-community/

Mears, S. (2017). It takes a community to raise a reader: Autism friendly libraries. http://library.ifla.org/1744/1/138-mears-en.pdf

Milestones Autism Resources. (2020). Self-advocacy & self-determination: How to share your needs and protect your rights. https://www.milestones.org/get-started/for-individuals/self-advocacy

Miller, L. K. (1999). The savant syndrome: Intellectual impairment and exceptional skill. *Psychological Bulletin*, 125(1), 31–46. doi:10.1037/0033-2909.125.1.31

Monteiro, M. (2016). *Family therapy and the autism spectrum: autism conversations in narrative practice.* Routledge.

National Alliance on Mental Illness (NAMI). (2020). Autism. https://www.nami.org/Learn-More/Mental-Health-Conditions/Related-Conditions/Autism

National Autism Association. (2012). Lethal outcomes in autism spectrum disorders (ASD) wandering/elopement. https://nationalautismassociation.org/wp-content/uploads/2012/01/Lethal-Outcomes-In-Autism-Spectrum-Disorders_2012.pdf

National Institute of Mental Health. (2020). Autism spectrum disorder. https://www.nimh.nih.gov/health/topics/autism-spectrum-disorders-asd/index.shtml

Obrey, E. (2019, June 14). Train the presenter training, [Presentation] Autism Friendly Training, Springfield, MO.

Obrey, E., & Barboa, L. (2015). *Tic toc autism clock: A guide to your 24/7 plan.* Goldminds Publishing.

Oesch, T. (2019, August 19). Autism at work: Hiring and training employees on the spectrum. *SHRM*. https://www.shrm.org/resourcesandtools/hr-topics/behavioral-competencies/global-and-cultural-effectiveness/pages/autism-at-work-hiring-and-training-employees-on-the-spectrum.aspx

Panzano, L. (2018). Five research-based strengths associated with autism. *Stages Learning Materials.* https://blog.stageslearning.com/blog/five-research-based-strengths-associated-with-autism

Povey, C. (2014, December 16). What is autism and why is public understanding important? *Independent.* https://www.independent.co.uk/life-style/health-and-families/features/what-autism-and-why-public-understanding-important-9927778.html

Prelock, P. (2006). *Autism spectrum disorders.* Pro-ed.

Reichow, B., & Volkmar, F. R. (2010). Social skills interventions for individuals with autism: Evaluation for evidence-based practices within a best evidence synthesis framework. *Journal of Autism and Developmental Disorders*, 40, 149–166.

Resnik, D. (2016). Lessons learned: Building the most autism friendly city in the world. *First Place Phoenix.* https://www.firstplaceaz.org/blog/lessons-learned-building-the-most-autism-friendly-city-in-the-world/

Rodden, J. (2020). What does autism spectrum disorder look like in adults? *Attitude* https://www.additudemag.com/autism-spectrum-disorder-in-adults/

Rosenblatt, A. I., & Carbone, P. S. (2019). *Autism spectrum disorder.* American Academy of Pediatrics.

Russell, G., Kapp, S. K., Elliott, D., Elphick, C., Gwernan-Jones, R., & Owens, C. (2019). Mapping the autistic advantage from the accounts of adults diagnosed with autism: A qualitative study. *Autism in Adulthood*, 1(2). 124–133 doi:10.1089/aut.2018.0035

Selfe, L. (2013). *Autism spectrum disorder.* McGraw-Hill.

Shattuck, P.T., Roux, A. M., Hudson, L. E., Taylor, J. L., Maenner, M. J., & Trani, J-F. (2012). Services for adults with an autism spectrum disorder. *The Canadian Journal of Psychiatry*, 57 (5), 284–291. doi:10.1177/070674371205700503

Shore, S. (2003). *Beyond the wall: Personal experiences with autism and Asperger Syndrome. Shawnee Mission.* Autism Asperger Publishing Company.

Sicile-Kira, C. (2004). *Autism spectrum disorders: The complete guide to understanding autism, Asperger's Syndrome, pervasive developmental disorder, and other ASDs.* Berkley Publishing Group.

Siri, K., & Lyons, T. (2010). *Cutting edge therapies for autism.* Skyhorse Publishing.

Stebbins, L. (2016). Five ways we can make the world more autism friendly. *Stages Learning Materials.* http://blog.stageslearning.com/blog/5-ways-we-can-make-the-world-more-autism-friendly

Stelter, L. (2018, April 2). Improving response to emergencies involving autistic children. American Military University. https://www.ems1.com/autism/articles/improving-response-to-emergencies-involving-autistic-children-zjbQkvpZTOwFH1Ah/

StopBullying.gov. (2020). Bullying and children and youth with disabilities and special health needs. https://www.stopbullying.gov/sites/default/files/2017-09/bullyingtipsheet.pdf

Swetlitz, I. (2017, February 27). Dimmed lights, loosened rules: Growing number of businesses cater to autistic visitors. *STAT.* https://www.statnews.com/2017/02/22/autism-shops-movies/

Syriopoulou-Delli, C. K., Agaliotis, I., & Papaefstathiou, E. (2018). Social skills characteristics of students with autism spectrum disorder. *International Journal of Developmental Disabilities.* 64 (1).

Turner, L. (2020, August 1). How to make your store more autism-friendly. *CWB*https://cwb-online.co/how-to-make-your-store-more-autism-friendly/

University of California, Berkeley Web Access. (2020). What is "descriptive audio"? https://webaccess.berkeley.edu/ask-pecan/descriptive-audio

University of Southern California (USC) Libraries. (2020). Preparing for your presentation. https://libguides.usc.edu/writingguide/oralpresentation

Vaughan, A. (2014). *Positively sensory! A guide to help your child develop positive approaches to learning and cope with sensory processing difficulty.* Scribble Media.

Vormer, C. (2020). *Connecting with the autism spectrum: How to talk, how to listen, and why you shouldn't call it high functioning.* Rockridge Press.

White House Archives. (2015). Barack Obama, Presidential Proclamation. https://obamawhitehouse.archives.gov/the-press-office/2015/04/01/presidential-proclamation-world-autism-awareness-day-2015

Wikipedia. (2020). Autism friendly. https://en.wikipedia.org/wiki/Autismfriendly

Winchester, S. (2011, May 28). A verb for our frantic times. *The New York Times.* https://www.nytimes.com/2011/05/29/opinion/29winchester.html

Wolfberg, P. (1999). *Play and imagination in children with autism.* Teachers College Press.

Index

Page numbers in italics refer to figures. Page numbers in bold refer to tables.

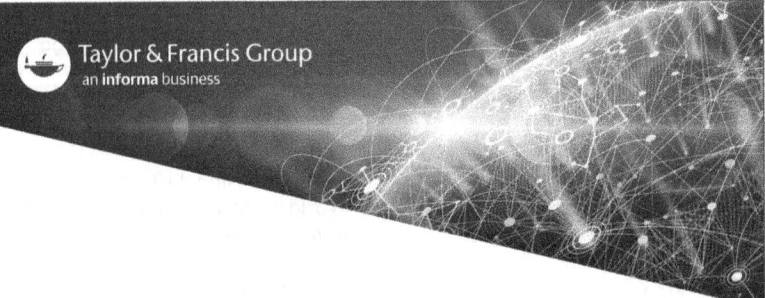
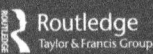
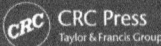